the**facts**

Pulmonary arterial hypertension

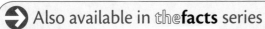

Also available in the**facts** series

the**facts**

Pulmonary arterial hypertension

DR CLIVE HANDLER BSc, MD, MRCP, FACC, FESC

Consultant in Pulmonary Hypertension,
Royal Free Hospital

Honorary Senior Lecturer,
UCL Medical School

Honorary Consultant Cardiologist,
Guy's and St Thomas' Hospitals

DR GERRY COGHLAN MD, FRCP

Consultant Cardiologist, Royal Free Hospital

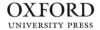

OXFORD
UNIVERSITY PRESS

OXFORD

UNIVERSITY PRESS

Great Clarendon Street, Oxford OX2 6DP

Oxford University Press is a department of the University of Oxford.
It furthers the University's objective of excellence in research, scholarship,
and education by publishing worldwide in

Oxford New York

Auckland Cape Town Dar es Salaam Hong Kong Karachi
Kuala Lumpur Madrid Melbourne Mexico City Nairobi
New Delhi Shanghai Taipei Toronto

With offices in

Argentina Austria Brazil Chile Czech Republic France Greece
Guatemala Hungary Italy Japan Poland Portugal Singapore
South Korea Switzerland Thailand Turkey Ukraine Vietnam

Oxford is a registered trade mark of Oxford University Press
in the UK and in certain other countries

Published in the United States
by Oxford University Press Inc., New York

British Library Cataloguing in Publication Data

Data available

Library of Congress Cataloging in Publication Data

Typeset in Plantin by Glyph International, Bangalore, India
Printed in Great Britain
on acid-free paper
by Ashford colour press

ISBN 978–0–19–958292–1

10 9 8 7 6 5 4 3 2 1

Whilst every effort has been made to ensure that the contents of this book are as complete, accurate
and up-to-date as possible at the date of writing, Oxford University Press is not able to give any
guarantee or assurance that such is the case. Readers are urged to take appropriately qualified
medical advice in all cases. The information in this book is intended to be useful to the general
reader, but should not be used as a means of self-diagnosis or for the prescription of medication.

Dr Clive Handler dedicates this book to his wife Caroline and their three children, Charlotte, Sophie, and Julius.

Dr Gerry Coghlan dedicates this book to his wife Eveleen and their three sons, Niall, Cathal, and Eoin.

About the Authors

Dr Clive Handler BSc, MD, MRCP, FACC, FESC is Consultant in Pulmonary Hypertension to The National Pulmonary Hypertension Unit at The Royal Free Hospital, London, Honorary Consultant Cardiologist to Guy's and St Thomas' Hospitals, Honorary Senior Lecturer in Medicine at UCL Medical School, and Consultant Cardiologist at The Hospital of St John and St Elizabeth, and Highgate Hospitals, London. He was previously Consultant Cardiologist at Northwick Park and St Mary's Hospitals, London. He trained at Guy's Hospital Medical School and at St Luke's Hospital Milwaukee, University of Wisconsin. He edited "Guy's Hospital—250 years" in 1975. His textbook "Cardiology in Primary Care", was published by Radcliffe Publishing in 2004. He is co-editor of "Classic Papers in Coronary Angioplasty" with Dr Michael Cleman from Yale University Medical School (Springer), and co-editor of "Vascular Complications in Human Disease: mechanisms and consequences", and "Advances in Vascular Medicine", both published by Springer, with Professor David Abraham, Dr Mick Dashwood and Dr Gerry Coghlan. Together with Dr Gerry Coghlan, he wrote "Management of Cardiac Problems in Primary Care, 2nd Edition", "Preventing Cardiovascular Disease in Primary Care, 2nd Edition", (Radcliffe Publishing), "Living with Coronary Disease" (Springer), and the Oxford Handbook of Pulmonary Hypertension. Together with Charlotte Handler and Dr Deborah Gill, he is the author of "English and reflective writing skills in medicine" (Radcliffe Publishing). He has written numerous scientific papers.

Dr Gerry Coghlan MD, FRCP is Consultant Cardiologist and Director of the National Pulmonary Hypertension Unit at the Royal Free Hospital. He trained in Dublin and at Harefield and the Royal Free Hospitals. He is an international authority on Pulmonary Arterial Hypertension and has wide interests in all aspects of the management of coronary heart disease and angioplasty. He has written several books with Dr Clive Handler as well as scientific papers on pulmonary hypertension and other aspects of cardiology.

Foreword

This book is essential for any patient who has recently been diagnosed with Pulmonary Arterial Hypertension.

In 1972 I was a mining engineer in Zambia, and had been suffering through many months of illness and the accompanying endless tests and procedures. When I was admitted to the mine hospital, a muscle biopsy confirmed that I had a connective tissue disease called dermatomyositis. I was given a high dose of steroids and when I was well enough I flew home. After this bad medical experience, I resolved to live my life to the full and not let the disease stop me. Happily, in 1992, I was taken off the small amount of medication I was taking and was told I was in remission. I was well aware of my good luck, and appreciated the good health I was in.

In 1979, I started working in Aviation as a non-destructive testing engineer, a job that involved a lot of physical activity, inspecting entire airplanes, both inside and out, for defects, corrosion, and damage.

Ominously, in 1999, I started feeling breathless when climbing up to perform an inspection of the tail of a 747 or a DC10. My daily job tasks were becoming difficult, or impossible, and eventually I had to stop working. Even after being referred to a consultant, I was frustrated at the lack of progress in finding out what was responsible for my breathlessness. I asked for a second opinion.

I was sent to The Royal Brompton Hospital in London. After another consultation, endless questions, and a whole series of tests, I was told that I possibly had Pulmonary Arterial Hypertension (PAH), and I was referred to the PAH Clinic at The Royal Free, who have an extensive experience of connective tissue diseases. I have now been a PAH patient at The Royal Free Hospital for about ten years.

Reading *Pulmonary Arterial Hypertension: The Facts* reminded me of my feelings at the time I was diagnosed; I was depressed and angry, feeling singled out to suffer from such a condition. My whole world had changed. I went from being an incredibly active person to someone who was physically very limited. Simple tasks like getting dressed and walking up stairs meant I had to pace myself in order to avoid being overcome by severe breathlessness.

PAH totally changed my outlook on life. Things that I once considered important now pale into insignificance; being able to do things and remain active take precedence over everything. I can fight my dermatomysitis with pain killers Trying to physically fight against my PAH results in breathlessness, followed by light-headedness, and blackouts.

A decade later, with medications regime including treprostinil and sildenafil, I am much improved. When I had my first cardiac catheter examination it was a relief just to find out the cause of my symptoms as I had been ill for nearly two years. It is a shock to be told you have an illness like PAH, but from my first appointment I have appreciated the support, openness and friendliness of the PAH Clinic. Now, additionally, I have the information in this very helpful and easy-to-read book, written by experts who understand patients and their concerns and anxieties. When I was first told I had PAH, I wanted to know more. Most people today will seek information on the internet; some of the web sites about PAH are, unfortunately and inaccurately sensationalist and quite frightening. Eventually, I joined PHA-UK and met more people with PAH. By talking with other patients on similar medication I found help, advice, and support.

Pulmonary Arterial Hypertension: The Facts explains what PAH is simply and factually. It details the diagnostic procedures, treatments, and the significant progress made with new drugs and research. This book is very informative, very positive, and it has given me hope, that even as a PAH veteran, I can continue to live as normally as possible with PAH. I'm quite sure it will do the same for others who are diagnosed with PAH.

Many thanks go to Drs Handler and Coghlan for writing this book, and for asking me to write a Foreword for it.

John Hayward, PAH patient, London, UK

Preface

Pulmonary arterial hypertension (PAH) is a not a new disease. The recent rapid and encouraging advances in our understanding of why and in whom it occurs, coupled with the arrival of several new treatments which improve quality of life and survival, have fuelled interest in early detection and treatment of this complex and serious disease. Early diagnosis depends on increased awareness, and this is fundamental to improving outcomes for patients with PAH.

Thirty years ago, when prostaglandins—drugs which act mainly by relaxing tense lung arteries—were the only available treatment, life expectancy and quality of life were abysmal. A diagnosis of PAH had similar implications to a diagnosis of some bad cancers. The outlook was so disappointing and dispiriting to patients, doctors, and nurses that there seemed little point in even pursuing the diagnosis. Doctors may have thought that even if they found that a patient's breathlessness was due to PAH, little could be done.

Very little was known about PAH. We still do not know why the lung arteries become thickened and narrowed. These changes lead to reduced blood flow to the lungs with reduced oxygen uptake in the blood. The most common symptoms are breathlessness, tiredness, and fatigue, and in severe cases, feeling faint or losing consciousness during exertion. Without effective treatment, the arterial changes can progress quite rapidly and the lung arteries become narrower. The resistance to blood flow through the lungs increases to a very high level, putting a strain on the right heart pumping chamber which eventually fails. When things get this bad, patients eventually die of heart failure.

The precise cause and mechanisms for the narrowing and thickening of the lung arteries are not known. Therefore a cure for PAH is not yet available. However, compared with 30 years ago, patients are now detected earlier, are seen by PAH specialists in specialist centres, receive an accurate diagnosis and characterization (there are several different conditions associated with or causing PAH) of their condition, and are being treated effectively. PAH drugs result in a better quality of life, and in most cases a longer life.

However, for some patients with severe PAH, this is clearly not enough. Their lives are blighted and their ability to lead an active and productive life is considerably restricted. Despite multiple drugs, they remain very breathless and tired, and are often unable to lead an independent life as they are tied to their home and dependent on oxygen.

This is very distressing for patients, their families and friends, their carers, and the medical and nursing staff. The medical management of these patients is complex and demanding, and requires great skill and experience from a multi-disciplinary team of doctors, nurses, pharmacists, and physiotherapists. At least as important are the patient's family, friends, carers, and a variety of other people. The patient is the centre of this close support team and, despite the stresses and strains and emotional and physical turmoil, has to do their best to just keep going. There really is no other way to do it or say it.

This bleak, tragic, and frightening picture is one end of the spectrum of patients with PAH. At the other end are many patients who have no, or almost no, symptoms. They lead a full and active life—they work, have a family, and pursue their career, hobbies, sports, and social activities. Looking at them, they appear completely normal. These patients are probably on tablets for their PAH and may be on other medication. They are closely monitored by their PAH specialists and nursing team every few months. Fortunately, because of a greater awareness of PAH and different forms of treatment, this type of patient is becoming more common. This is the main aim of treating PAH—to allow patients to live as normal and as long a life as possible. This is really good news and encouraging to everyone involved with or touched by PAH.

We believe that explaining all aspects of PAH to patients, their families, and their carers is a fundamental part of high-quality medical and nursing care. Usually, the more patients understand about their condition, the easier they cope with it. Most patients want to know 'Why me and what is going to happen to me?'

We have written this book principally to help patients, their families, and their carers, but also everyone involved in managing these patients. We have tried to give this information in a straightforward, direct, factual, and where possible, reassuring and encouraging way. Because we do not know all the answers yet, we have also been frank about the areas of doubt and where there are holes in our knowledge.

PAH affects people of all ages, both children and adults. We are specialists in managing adult PAH and so we have not included the very specialist management of PAH in children.

When the condition deteriorates, we have to explain the possible consequences. Sadly, as in many other areas of medicine, there is no way to avoid confronting these very difficult and sad issues. Patients and their families understand that although they bear the burden of PAH, we are all in it together, working together with one clear objective—to improve our understanding of all aspects of this condition and to try to find its cause and its cure.

There is much work to do, and we all need determination and perseverance. The results from clinical trials of new treatments, and the outcomes from registries of patients followed up in specialist centres, are the cornerstones of our continually improving knowledge. Working with government agencies, we aim to give each patient the best treatment. Considerable progress is being made in all aspects of diagnosis and treatment and we are pleased that patient outcomes are improving. Where there was darkness, there is now light and justified optimism.

Clive Handler

Gerry Coghlan

The National Pulmonary Hypertension Unit

Royal Free Hospital, London

Acknowledgements

We are grateful to the PHA-UK for their support and endorsement of this book.

We are very grateful to our wonderful senior specialist nurse colleagues, pharmacists, commissioning managers and administrative staff, who work closely with us providing a superb, highly professional, and expert service to our patients.

We are indebted to Professor Dame Carol Black who established the Royal Free Scleroderma and Pulmonary Hypertension Unit. We would also like to thank Professor Christopher Denton and Dr Geraldine Brough, and our excellent registrars and research fellows, who work closely with us in the joint scleroderma and PAH service at the Royal Free Hospital.

Professor David Abraham and his team from UCL are a constant inspiration to us in all our academic and research endeavours.

We are grateful to our colleagues in the Pulmonary Hypertension Physicians group for their support.

We are grateful to Julius Handler who proof-read the manuscript.

Finally, and most importantly, we could not, and would not, have written this book without the continual inspiration from our patients who teach us so much every day.

Contents

Abbreviations

CTED-PAH	chronic thromboembolic disease associated pulmonary arterial hypertension
CTPA	contrast-enhanced computed tomographic pulmonary angiography
DVT	deep vein thrombosis
ERA	endothelin receptor antagonist
FPAH	familial pulmonary arterial hypertension
HRCT	high-resolution computed tomography
IPAH	idiopathic pulmonary arterial hypertension
MRI	magnetic resonance imaging
PAH	pulmonary arterial hypertension
PCT	primary care trust
PDE-5	phosphodiesterase-5
PHA	Pulmonary Hypertension Association

1

So you've been told you have pulmonary arterial hypertension (PAH)

➡ Key points

◆ PAH is a rare complex condition of unknown cause.

◆ It is very difficult to predict how the condition will affect individual patients and how they will respond to treatment.

◆ It is important that patients discuss their problems with their PAH team.

◆ The outlook for patients with PAH has improved considerably recently.

◆ Understanding PAH and how it affects the heart usually makes it easier for patients and their families to cope.

◆ PAH should be considered as a cause of breathlessness which is not explained by other more common conditions.

📄 Lauren's story

Lauren arrived in at school at 8 a.m. as usual. She was a busy school teacher and it was summer exam time. Her husband, Peter, had taken the two children, Alex aged 9 and Jenny aged 7, to their school on his way to work in the local bank. He was a good husband and a good father. Lauren and Peter had been together since college and had been married for 12 years.

Lauren was worried and was becoming more concerned about herself. She had not gone to the gym for months. This was partly because of her extra school duties, but she had been also found it increasingly difficult to exercise and do housework. She felt tired and breathless doing even light housework and shopping. She was not her usual sparky self.

Today she was going to find out what was wrong with her. She was going to see a consultant who specialized in pulmonary arterial hypertension (PAH). She was worried.

Until a year ago, she had been fit, going to the gym twice a week and swimming three times a week with the children. She took school netball and gym lessons, and passed on her love of exercise and sport to her children and pupils. She had told Peter that she was getting tired and breathless. Her father's serious illness had depressed her psychologically and physically. Peter initially thought that it was because she was overstretched at work. Lauren did not agree. She had gone to see her GP when she started to feel unwell. The GP told her that looking after young energetic children and holding down a full-time busy teaching job were more than enough to explain why she felt exhausted. The GP did not think there was anything serious for her to worry about.

Month by month, Lauren found it more difficult doing housework and cycling to school. Three months later she went back to see her GP who now thought she might have asthma. She was prescribed some inhalers but these did not help. Lauren had never smoked, was a slim 38-year-old happily married outgoing woman, who loved her family, and enjoyed her job. She and Peter socialized with friends at weekends and enjoyed their annual camping summer holiday.

Lauren was getting worse. She tried to do some exercises in the gym but could barely walk on the treadmill. She could hardly make the beds and found herself getting exhausted doing light housework. She went back to tell her GP, who referred her urgently to the chest physician at her local hospital.

After a thorough examination, the specialist told her that there was probably nothing to worry about, but that she may have become unfit through not exercising as intensely as before. The specialist ordered some tests including a chest X-ray, an electrical recording of the heart (ECG), some blood tests, breathing tests (lung function), and a heart ultrasound scan (echocardiogram). Lauren knew that something was not right but she could not understand what it was.

The day after the tests had been completed, the chest specialist's secretary phoned her. They wanted Lauren to return to clinic the following week. Lauren was anxious and worried. The chest specialist told her that although the chest X-ray and blood tests were normal, the heart ultrasound scan was abnormal, showing that the pressure in the lung arteries was high—a condition called pulmonary arterial hypertension (PAH). The breathing tests were also abnormal, showing a reduction in the ability of the lungs to transfer gases across from the air sac to the blood. He told her that this was a very rare and serious condition. Because he was not an expert in this condition, he wanted to refer her to a PAH specialist.

Lauren then looked up PAH on the Internet and cried. She cried when her neighbour dropped the children off after school. She cried when Peter came home after work. She cried nearly all week.

She went to her clinic appointment at the specialist PAH unit and tried to take in what the doctors and nurses told her. She was told that, based on the heart ultrasound, she probably did have PAH but a special heart catheter test was necessary to confirm or exclude the diagnosis. No other test could answer the question of whether she had PAH or not.

Shortly after the clinic appointment, she was admitted as a day case. Under local anaesthetic, a small thin tube was passed through a vein, through the right heart, and then into the lung arteries. The tube allowed measurements to be taken in the heart and lungs. The procedure was painless and took less than half an hour. While doing the test, the consultant told her that the test confirmed that she had PAH and that she would need tablets.

Before Peter picked her up from the hospital, Lauren spent time with the specialist PAH nurses who explained things again and arranged for her to come back to the PAH clinic the following week for her tablets. All the staff were very nice, patient, sympathetic, friendly, and very helpful. They explained things simply without rushing and gave her their helpline telephone number and an appointment date for her and her husband to come to the clinic the following week to discuss things further. Lauren felt reassured and 'looked after' and less scared. She understood that PAH was a serious condition but knew she was in the best possible hands. She felt that she could now cope with this condition and could rely on the staff at the PAH unit to give her the best treatments, advice, and support.

Lauren went back to work but reduced her teaching commitments. She is doing well, has gone back to the gym to do light exercises, and has stabilized on her medications.

Lessons from the case history

This case history is not unusual. It highlights several features about PAH.

◆ It affects young women more often than men. The reasons for this are unclear.

◆ There is often a time delay of at least a year before it is diagnosed. This is because PAH is rare, and doctors are trained to think of much more common conditions before considering rare or unusual diseases as a cause of a patient's symptoms. This is why the GP thought that Lauren may have been tired or unfit, or may have had asthma. These are much more common than PAH.

♦ Heart ultrasound and breathing tests (lung function) are very helpful in detecting people who may have PAH. However, both tests may be normal in people with mild PAH. Lung function is usually normal or very mildly affected in PAH, but the test is very helpful in finding other causes of breathlessness. If both tests are normal, this means PAH and serious lung problems are unlikely.

♦ The ECG is usually helpful but the changes due to PAH can be mistaken for other conditions. Like a chest X-ray, it may be normal unless the patient has severe PAH with damage to the right heart pumping chamber.

♦ Patients with suspected PAH should be referred to a specialist centre as soon as possible so that the diagnosis can be confirmed or excluded and advice given by a multidisciplinary team of experts. This requires awareness of the condition.

♦ A heart catheter test (a small tube called a catheter inserted into a vein in the groin or neck) is necessary to confirm that the patient has, or has not got, PAH. It is generally safe and harmless. Around 1 in 2000 patients may have a serious problem, such as heart rhythm disturbance or damage to the leg or neck vessels during or shortly after the procedure. The test also provides other information on the type and severity of the PAH and how well the heart is working. If it is necessary to see if a patient has blockages or narrowing in the heart arteries, a different tube is inserted into the artery in the groin to inject contrast fluid into the heart arteries. This is called a coronary angiogram. Both tests are done at the same time.

♦ Most patients with PAH are treated with tablets, at least initially.

Shock, fear, and confusion

You and your family may be in a state of shock and may be very worried and confused about what you have been told. You may even not believe that you have PAH.

Some people, particularly fit young people who have been diagnosed early, may feel pretty normal even though they have high blood pressure in their lungs. This is probably because the right side of the heart is coping with the high pressure in the lungs.

Other PAH patients may have noticed increasing breathlessness, fatigue, lack of energy, and other symptoms. These patients may have mixed emotions about being told that they have PAH. They are relieved that at last a cause has been found, having previously been thought to be neurotic, tired, stressed, or have a rare form of asthma. However, they now know that PAH is a serious and complex condition.

The severity of symptoms varies a lot between people even if they have a similar pressure in their lung arteries. Some feel fine and can do most things with only minimal limitation. Others become breathless doing light housework or walking a few hundred yards. No two patients are the same. No two patients respond in the same way to medications.

> The key thing is that you are in good hands. You should remember that your PAH team are experts in treating PAH. They understand your anxieties and fears and want to do everything they can to help, advise, and support you. You will get the best treatment. You are not alone.

Coping with PAH

Stay calm and do not panic. Although pulmonary arterial hypertension is a complex condition of unknown cause, and even difficult to pronounce (and that is why we shorten it to PAH), all is not lost. Over the last few years there have been considerable advances in our knowledge about PAH. Importantly, there are several new treatments which have improved the outlook for patients with PAH.

Advances in research and new medications

There are continuing advances in research into how and why PAH occurs. There are several trials of new treatments. These will help us decide which new treatments offer advantages and will make a difference to our patients. We are grateful to patients who agree to participate in clinical trials. Over the last few years several new drugs have become available, and more drugs are coming on stream every year. We are now treating more patients with more than one type of tablet for PAH if we feel it necessary for their particular case. We call this combination treatment—two or more different types of medication combined. We tailor treatment to the individual.

Survival of patients with PAH has steadily improved over the last 10 years. We hope that, with the results of research into the cause of PAH and trials of new medications, survival and quality of life for PAH patients will continue to improve.

Optimism and hope

So although there is not yet a cure for PAH, many doctors and researchers around the world are working together, very hard, to find the cause and cure. Compared with the rather desperate and depressing state of affairs in the 1990s, when there was only one type of treatment (prostacyclin), there are now several types of treatment. Patients are living longer and more productive lives. There is justified cause for optimism and hope.

Why you should not believe everything you read in the press or on the Internet

Much of the information about PAH on the Internet is frightening and out of date, and some of it is simply not true. It is very difficult, if not impossible, to obtain clear, accurate, and understandable information that is *relevant to your particular case* from the Internet or elsewhere. The best you can get from even a good Internet site is generalized advice.

As with any information site, newspaper or magazine article, or TV or radio programme, it is important to know when it was written, who wrote it, and whether they are experts. Do they really know what they are talking about? Not all doctors are experts in PAH.

This is particularly relevant when it comes to newspaper articles. The report may refer to a recent research publication or conference. These reports should be read with caution. Although there are knowledgeable and responsible journalists in various fields, medical and health issues are generally not covered accurately or in a balanced way unless they are written by medical experts. Health issues in certain newspapers and magazines are generally sensationalist and, unfortunately, alarmist. Articles may be fed to journalists from a public relations firm promoting an individual's or company's vested interest.

Journalists write in a very different way from medical researchers, who describe the details of what they have done and why, what they have discovered, and then discuss both the strengths and weaknesses of their study, and put their findings in the context of other studies. Journalists usually pick up a point from a press release and then expand on it if they think it is of interest or controversial. It may not even be the main point, or even true! It is just something that the journalist thinks will startle the reader.

Journalists are not doctors (although a few doctors do write newspaper columns occasionally), and very few journalists are trained scientists. However, they have a responsibility to write honestly and in a balanced way and report facts. There is no requirement for accuracy or balance when providing their opinion or reporting someone else's opinion. Even though they should seek expert advice on certain topics, this is very unusual. At best, they might include a very brief comment from a spokesperson from a medical organization or charity.

Whereas scientific and medical papers are 'peer reviewed' (checked and criticized, and changed if necessary before publication), newspaper articles are usually written to tight deadlines with little checking or verification. Inaccuracies, half-truths, 'spin', or nuances which distort or give an unbalanced view can frighten or worry patients and their families. The aim of the article is to make an impact on the reader. A patient's shock, worry, or false hope concerning 'miracle cures', 'superfoods', 'wonder drugs', and 'life-saving operations' is the patient's problem, not the responsibility of the journalist or the newspaper. Patients either look for more information from a patient support group or, more commonly, see their GP.

As busy clinicians, we bump into this situation often. Patients bring torn-out articles from a newspaper or a print-out from the Internet.

'Doctor, what do you think of this?'

'This article says that if I eat …, my PAH will go away.'

'There is a new wonder tablet which cures PAH. Can I have it?'

'Should I be on this tablet which has these awful side-effects or causes ….?'

'There is a story of a patient with PAH who has terrible trouble. Will I get to be like that?'

These are consequences of bad journalism and there is little we can do about it. Doctors have to deal with this and reassure patients' journalist-induced fears and anxieties with careful explanations. Patients should read as much as they want, but should not believe everything they read, unless they read accurate information from a reliable source. A healthy intelligent scepticism is helpful.

We are all unique

 The way you respond to your PAH, and any other associated medical condition you may have, is likely to be different from other people with the same condition.

Consider the different ways people react to stress, a cold, flu, indigestion, backache, or medications. Some people are very ill and take a long time to recover; others are hardly affected or recover overnight. Some people have side-effects from drugs, while most do not. The same condition affects each of us in a different way because each person has a different response to the same physical or emotional upset.

The reasons for these variations are complex and unknown. An example is an uncommon skin and gut condition called scleroderma, the cause of which is not known. Why some people with scleroderma get PAH and others may also get lung scarring, while most scleroderma patients do not, is unknown and is the subject of active research.

Problems in predicting the future

PAH patients and their families understandably want to know about their future, particularly if they have read or have been told worrying things about PAH.

Some patients want to know how long they will live. Of course, we are not able to answer this question accurately.

We try to address patients' concerns and anxieties and tell them how they are doing based on clinical examinations, the results of their tests, and the cardiac catheter findings. We can tell them if they are improving, stable, or deteriorating compared with their previous test results. But we are unable to tell them how long they will live.

There are many things we do not know about PAH. Because each patient is unique and responds in a different way to their illness and treatments, we cannot predict the future for one patient from the outcome in a different patient even if they have the same type of PAH. We can, at best, give them only a very approximate and often meaningless answer. We simply just cannot guess it correctly. Crystal ball gazing in medicine is a very dangerous pursuit. It is like tossing a coin—as often wrong as right—and therefore unhelpful.

 Patients usually know when they are stable or doing well, and also know if they are not.

Patient support groups and charities

The patient group websites are helpful. They provide background information, practical advice to patients and their families, and also carry out political lobbying and provide a voice for patients.

 Probably the best and most helpful source of information is from your PAH specialist clinical team who is looking after you. They will give you accurate and up-to-date information that is relevant to you because they know your case better than anyone else.

Specialist PAH centres

PAH is rare. Like other rare medical conditions, patients with PAH are usually treated in large hospitals where there are teams of clinical specialists who have extensive experience and expertise in diagnosing, managing, and advising patients with PAH. Large hospitals have up-to-date investigation equipment, scanning services, and cardiac testing services.

PAH centres in the UK are 'recognized' as specialist centres by the Government. This allows them to prescribe treatments for PAH, which currently are expensive, costing tens of thousands of pounds per patient per year. These treatments can be only be prescribed by recognized PAH specialists.

There are seven recognized PAH centres in England: Newcastle, Sheffield, Brompton Hospital, Papworth Hospital, Hammersmith Hospital, Great Ormond Street Hospital for Children, and the Royal Free Hospital. There is also one in Dublin and one in Glasgow. Some of the units have a particular interest and expertise in a particular type of PAH. For example, Papworth Hospital is the only hospital in the UK where patients can go to have an operation to remove large blood clots (pulmonary emboli) from lung arteries. This operation is called thromboendarterectomy and can be very helpful for suitable patients. At the Royal Free Hospital we specialize in PAH associated with connective tissue diseases. Great Ormond Street Hospital is a major children's hospital and naturally specializes in congenital PAH affecting children.

The centres work collaboratively, and the clinicians meet formally at least twice a year to discuss how the service nationally can be improved and developed. There are joint research meetings so that they can learn from each other. They also meet health managers from the Department of Health who commission PAH services to audit, plan, develop, and improve these services. Therefore PAH patients in the UK receive similar treatment and benefit from the experience and expertise of a large group of dedicated active PAH specialists. The PAH centres in the UK, and others from around the world, work together on clinical trials on new treatments. PAH has become a world community of patients and clinicians dedicated to improving the lives of patients with PAH.

PAH teams are multidisciplinary. This means that the team members have many different and complementary skills and expertise. Most PAH teams consist of specialist PAH consultants (cardiologists and/or respiratory physicians), senior nurse specialists, pharmacists, administrative staff, managers who are responsible for obtaining funding for the treatments, social workers, and, in some hospitals, counsellors.

PAH is often associated with other medical conditions. Other specialists, including rheumatologists (bone and joint experts), liver specialists, HIV specialists, haematologists (specialist in blood disorders), thoracic surgeons (who sometimes may consider it helpful to remove large blood clots which have blocked lung arteries), and transplant surgeons, are available in either the hospital or other centres to provide patients with all the necessary help.

Very often, patients are seen in joint clinics. For example, patients whose PAH is associated with a connective tissue disease are seen by a PAH specialist and a rheumatologist, as well as by other staff. This provides patients with a holistic approach.

Outreach centres

In many countries, including the UK, there are 'outreach clinics' where PAH specialists go to hospitals and work with other specialists in joint clinics. The PAH specialist can apply for PAH treatments on behalf of the local consultants.

Outreach clinics are convenient for patients who can see a PAH specialist at their local hospital and so do not need to travel long distances to a PAH centre.

The problems with a rare disease

PAH is rare. It is estimated to occur in around 20 in every million people. However, this may be an underestimate because some patients who have PAH may not be diagnosed. Therefore hardly any GPs, most of whom look after around 2000 patients, will ever see a PAH patient. Most heart or lung specialists will see perhaps one or two patients in their career.

The aims of this book

We hope that after reading this short book, you and your family will understand more about PAH. We believe that that the more you understand, the more easily you will cope with your condition. If you are a family member or friend of a patient, we hope that the information in this book will also help you understand more about PAH—what it is, how it is diagnosed and what tests are done and why, which medical conditions are linked to PAH (although PAH most commonly occurs on its own), the problems that PAH patients might encounter and how these are treated, and the types of treatments that we currently use. There is a lot more to PAH treatment than just tablets, injectable medicines, and oxygen. We will be covering all the aspects of treatment.

In order to understand PAH and how it affects the heart and lungs, it is helpful to understand the workings of the normal heart and lungs. We deal with this in the next chapter.

2

The structure of the heart

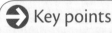 Key points

- The heart consists of two separate pumps joined side by side.
- The right and left sides of the heart pump at the same time.
- There are two separate but connected circulations.
- The right heart pumps used blood to the lungs where it picks up oxygen.
- The refreshed oxygenated blood travels to the left side of the heart.
- The left heart pumps oxygenated blood around the body.

Our special heart

The heart is essentially a pump, but a rather special one. No pump made by man could do the job our heart does. Nowadays, most people live for 80 years or more with the same heart with no need for repairs, oil changes, or new parts! The human heart has to pump blood around the body once a second, 60 times per minute. That is an astounding 3 billion beats during a 90 year life. Each heart beat consists of both a contraction and a relaxation phase. Blood is squeezed out of the pumping chambers during contaction (systole). The pumping chambers are refilled with blood when the muscle pump relaxes (diastole).

Our heart has to be able to increase the volume of blood it ejects on demand. When we exercise or move around, the muscles of our arms and legs need more blood, oxygen, and nutrients. This is achieved by the heart beating faster to deliver more blood around the body. It is similar to putting your foot on the accelerator pedal.

The volume of blood ejected or pumped out of the heart in a minute is called the cardiac output. The cardiac output may have to increase fivefold instantaneously if, for example, we have to run to catch a bus. Even the best supercar engine could not perform as well as that. The heart, being the size of an adult fist, is also considerably smaller than a car engine. This is why it is so important to look after our heart.

What does the heart look like?

The heart is a hard-working pump made of dark red muscle the size of an adult fist. It is shaped like a blunt-ended cone.

Where is the heart?

The heart is found just beneath and to the left of the breastbone (sternum). When we lean forward or lie on our left side, the heart falls against the rib cage. This is why people may feel their heartbeat (palpitation) when lying in bed.

The structure of the heart (Figure 2.1)

The heart consists of the following.

- Two pumps joined side by side but separated by a partition wall called the ventricular septum.

- There are four hollow chambers. The two pumping chambers are called the right and left ventricles. The two collecting or receiving chambers are called the right and left atria.

- The flow and direction of blood around the heart are controlled by four valves. There are two on the left side and two on the right side of the heart.

The left side of the heart

The left side of the heart consists of the following.

- A collecting chamber (left atrium) receives fresh oxygenated blood from the lungs.

- The mitral valve is situated between the left atrium and the left ventricle. When open, it allows blood to flow from the left atrium to the left ventricle. When closed, it prevents blood leaking back from the ventricle to the atrium when the ventricle contracts (squeezes).

- The left pumping chamber (left ventricle) pumps blood around the body. Its walls are much thicker than the right ventricle because it has to pump blood against a higher pressure and therefore has more work to do. The pressure in the arteries and smaller arteries (arterioles) of the body is normally much higher than the pressure in the lung (pulmonary) arteries. When the pressure in the arteries is high (hypertension), the wall of the left ventricle becomes thicker in order to generate sufficient pressure inside the pumping chamber to force blood around the system.

- The aortic valve (outflow valve) is situated between the left ventricle and the main arterial trunk called the aorta. When open, it allows blood to be ejected from the ventricle into the aorta for distribution around the body. When closed, it prevents ejected blood from leaking back from the aorta into the ventricle.

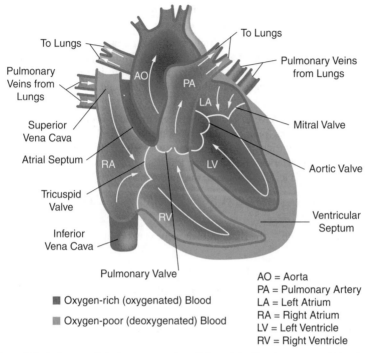

Figure 2.1 A diagram of the heart opened up. Light red signifies deoxygenated blood. Dark red indicates oxygenated blood. Deoxygenated blood returning from all parts of the body in the veins reaches the right atrium (RA). It passes through the tricuspid valve between the right atrium and the right ventricle. It is then pumped through the pulmonary valve to the pulmonary artery (PA) and to the lungs for oxygenation. The oxygenated blood returns to the left atrium (LA) and passes through the mitral valve into the left ventricle from where it is pumped through the aortic valve into the aorta (AO) and then around the body.

The right side of the heart

The right heart side of the heart consists of the following.

- The right collecting chamber (right atrium) receives stale blood, containing very little oxygen, from all parts of the body.

- The tricuspid (three cusps or leaflets) valve is situated between the right atrium and the right ventricle. When open, it allows blood flow from the right atrium to the right ventricle. When closed, it prevents blood leaking back from the ventricle to the atrium when the ventricle contracts. The tricuspid valve is the heart valve of most relevance to patients with PAH.

13

Ultrasound examination of blood flow across the tricuspid is helpful in estimating the pressure in the lung arteries.

◆ The right pumping chamber (right ventricle) pumps oxygen-poor blood to the lungs. The walls of the right ventricle are thin because it pumps blood into a low-pressure system. In PAH, the pressure in the lung arteries is increased. This can cause the right ventricle to become weak and fail, causing breathlessness.

◆ The pulmonary valve is situated between the right ventricle and the main artery to the lungs (pulmonary artery). When open, it allows blood to be ejected from the ventricle into the pulmonary artery for distribution around the lung arteries, arterioles (smaller lung arteries), and capillaries. When closed, it prevents blood leaking back from the pulmonary artery into the ventricle.

Do the right and left heart pumps pump and relax at the same time?

Yes. The two pumps—the right and left ventricles—contract together and relax together.

The heart cycle: systole (squeezing or contraction of the pumping chambers) and diastole (relaxation and filling of the pumping chambers)

◆ The phase when the heart pumps squeeze blood out of the pumping chambers (ventricles) is called systole.

◆ The phase when the heart pumps fill with blood from their collecting chambers (atria) is called diastole.

What is an artery?

An artery is a muscular-walled blood vessel supplying blood and oxygen to the organs of our body (Figure 2.2). All arteries, except the lung (pulmonary) arteries, carry oxygen-rich blood to every cell.

What is a vein?

A vein is a thin-walled non-muscular blood vessel carrying stale deoxygenated blood back to the right side of the heart (Figure 2.3). Veins have valves so that blood can return to the heart. When the valves are damaged, the pressure in the veins increases. The veins become fatter and more visible—'varicose veins'—and may leak blood and fluid. Veins are more visible and stand out more after exercise and in warm weather. They are less easily seen in cold weather.

All the blood from the arms, legs, skin, and abdomen return in veins to the right side of the heart. The small capillaries draining the organs join up to form larger and larger veins. The blood from the head, neck, and arms drains into a very large vein called the superior vena cava which drains into the upper part of the

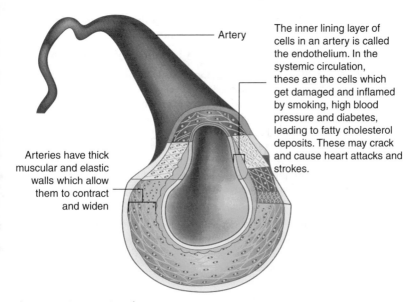

Artery

The inner lining layer of cells in an artery is called the endothelium. In the systemic circulation, these are the cells which get damaged and inflamed by smoking, high blood pressure and diabetes, leading to fatty cholesterol deposits. These may crack and cause heart attacks and strokes.

Arteries have thick muscular and elastic walls which allow them to contract and widen

Figure 2.2 Cross-section of an artery.

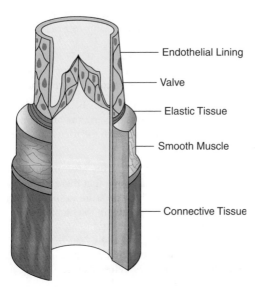

Endothelial Lining

Valve

Elastic Tissue

Smooth Muscle

Connective Tissue

Figure 2.3 Cross-section of a vein.

right atrium. The blood from the abdomen and legs drains into the inferior vena cava which drains into the lower part of the right atrium.

Blood samples are taken from veins, usually in the front of the elbow crease.

If a vein is cut, the bleeding can be stopped easily by pressing on the cut for a few minutes. This is because the pressure in veins is low—5mmHg (capable of pushing mercury up 5 mm against the force of gravity). Stopping bleeding from a cut artery is much more difficult because the pressure in an artery is 20 times higher (120mmHg) than that in a vein.

What is a pulmonary (lung) artery?

There is one main pulmonary artery leaving the right heart pumping chamber (right ventricle). This main 'trunk' divides into two—one to the right lung and one to the left lung.

The pulmonary arteries carry deoxygenated blood to the lungs for refreshment with oxygen. The lung vessels divide into progressively smaller blood vessels. The main pulmonary arteries are around 2–3 cm in diameter. The walls of the pulmonary arteries, like other arteries, contain elastic and muscle layers and an inner lining of endothelial cells.

In PAH the artery walls and the endothelial layer of cells become thickened and narrowed. This reduces the blood flow to the lungs, resulting in a low oxygen level in the blood. When a large proportion of the medium and small lung arteries are narrowed, the resistance to blood flow in the lungs increases. This causes high pressure in the lung arteries (PAH). The right ventricle has to work harder to pump blood against a high resistance and this causes right heart failure.

Jugular (neck) veins

There are four jugular veins, two on each side of the neck. They each drain blood from the head and neck into the right heart collecting chamber (right atrium).

The neck veins may be very prominent in PAH because of distension or swelling of the neck veins with blood. This is because the high pressure in the lungs is transmitted back to the right heart, through the tricuspid valve, and then back to the jugular veins.

Doctors examine the jugular veins to see if the pressure in the heart is high or low. A high pressure in the neck veins shows that there is a high pressure in the right atrium and ventricle due to a high pressure in the lung arteries. Patients with severe PAH often have a high pressure in the jugular veins.

Pulmonary veins

After passing through the millions of tiny capillaries in the lungs, oxygenated blood flows in four large pulmonary veins back to the left heart collecting chamber (left atrium).

3

The oxygenation and circulation of blood

→ Key points

- Blood circulates around the body in two parallel but connected circuits. These are the pulmonary (lung) circulation and the systemic circulation (all parts of the body except the lungs).
- The right heart pumps deoxygenated or stale blood to the lungs where it is refreshed with oxygen.
- The refreshed or oxygenated blood then circulates to the left heart.
- The left heart pumps oxygenated blood to all parts of the body.
- After supplying all the organs with oxygen, glucose, and other nutrients, the blood becomes deoxygenated.
- The deoxygenated blood circulates back to the right side of the heart in the veins.

The circulation of blood

What does 'circulation' mean?

Circulation is the flow of blood around the body. There are two parallel but connected circulations, one to the lungs and the other to the rest of the body (Figure 3.1).

'Parallel' means that the right side of the heart, pumping blood to the lungs, and the left side of the heart, pumping blood around the rest of the body, contract and relax at the same time.

'Connected' means that blood pumped to the lungs travels from the lungs to the left side of the heart.

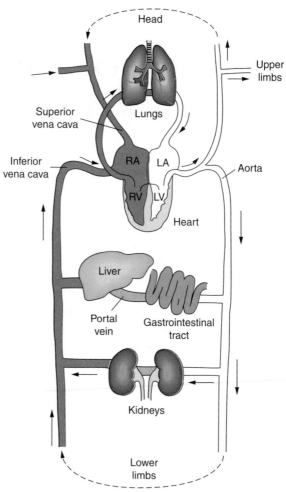

Figure 3.1 Diagram of the circulation of blood.

1. Stale blood, containing little oxygen, from all parts of the body (coloured grey) returns in blood vessels called veins to the right side of the heart. The main vein draining the abdomen (tummy) and legs is called the inferior vena cava because it enters the lower part of the right heart's collecting chamber (right atrium (RA)). The main vein draining the head, neck, and arms is called the superior vena cava because it enters the upper part of the right heart's collecting chamber.

2. The right heart pump (the right ventricle (RV)) then pumps this deoxygenated blood to the lungs.

Figure 3.1 (*continued*).

3. The stale deoxygenated blood picks up oxygen in the lungs from the air we breathe in.

4. The oxygen is carried around in the blood attached to a protein substance in the red blood cells called haemoglobin.

5. The fresh oxygenated blood (coloured white) then circulates (travels) to the left side of the heart in the pulmonary veins.

6. The left heart pump (the left ventricle (LV)) pumps oxygenated blood out through the main artery, called the aorta, to all parts of the body in blood vessels called arteries.

7. The fresh oxygenated blood supplies every cell in every organ of the body with oxygen, glucose, and nutrients, without which they cannot function and do their job.

8. The blood leaving the organs and limbs is now deoxygenated and returns to the right side of the heart.

Why is oxygenated blood bright red and deoxygenated blood dark blue?

Oxygen travels on a protein in the red cells called haemoglobin. When oxygen is attached to the protein, the blood cells look bright red. This is called oxygenated blood.

Oxygen is extracted (removed from) from the haemoglobin when the blood reaches the organs and cells. Red cells without oxygen look dark blue. This is called deoxygenated blood.

What do the lungs do and how are they related to the lung arteries?

The lungs are responsible for oxygenating the blood. The diaphragm is a muscle separating the chest from the abdomen. When it contracts, it enlarges the chest cavity (making the lungs larger), reducing the pressure in the lungs so that air is sucked into the chest. Air containing around 21% oxygen is breathed in and travels down large air tubes called bronchi. These divide into smaller and smaller tubes called bronchioles. The smallest air tubes become millions of tiny blind-ended hollow sacs, called alveoli which look rather like bunches of grapes (Figures 3.2 and 3.3).

Wrapped around the alveoli are capillaries. These are the smallest lung vessels. They are too small to be seen by the naked eye and so can only be seen using a powerful microscope. Their walls are one cell thick, and so oxygen and carbon dioxide, a waste gas formed as a by-product of metabolism, can pass in opposite directions across the capillary wall.

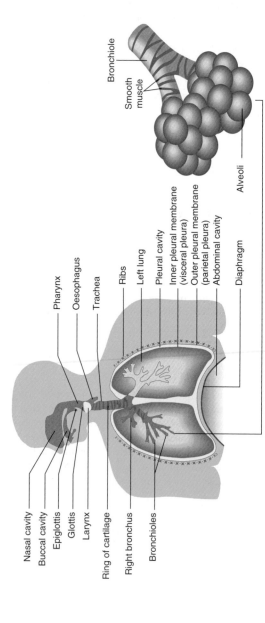

Figure 3.2 Diagram of the breathing parts of the mouth, neck, and chest. Air enters the nose and/or mouth and travels down the main air tube called the trachea. This divides into two main air tubes, the right bronchus and the left bronchus. These then divide into smaller and smaller air tubes before becoming very small closed air sacs called alveoli. Gas exchange takes place in the alveoli.

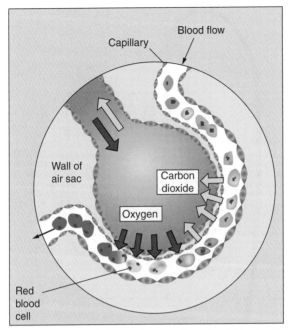

Figure 3.3 An alveolus, showing passage of oxygen (from the air breathed in) through the very thin capillary wall into the blood where it attaches to haemoglobin. Blood refreshed with oxygen is called oxygenated blood. It circulates from the lung to the left side of the heart, and from there to all parts of the body. Carbon dioxide is a waste product gas formed from metabolic processes in the cells and organs. It is carried in the blood from the organs via veins to the right side of the heart where it travels from the pulmonary arteries to the tiny capillaries in the lungs. It passes from the capillary across the membrane to the alveolus and is breathed out. Capillaries join up to form larger veins. These veins form four large lung (pulmonary) veins which carry oxygenated blood back to the left heart collecting chamber (left atrium).

How is the oxygen content of the blood measured?

Oxygen content is measured using a clip or oximeter placed over a finger nail or earlobe (Figure 3.4). A light sensor measures the brightness of the blood. The higher the oxygen content, the brighter the blood. The normal oxygen content is 96–99%. A more accurate but slightly painful method is to take a blood sample from an artery, most commonly the radial artery at the wrist. The oximeter is unreliable in recording the oxygen saturation in patients with scleroderma or other causes of bad circulation in the hands and fingers. In such cases a blood sample is taken from an artery, usually the artery in the groin (femoral artery),

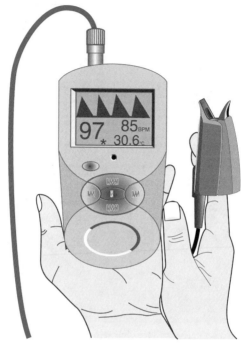

Figure 3.4 An oximeter for measuring the concentration of oxygen in the blood using a clip placed over a finger nail. The normal range is 96–99%. There are several reasons for a low reading.

and a catheter test is used to measure the pressures in the right heart and lung arteries.

Why might the oxygen content of the blood be low?

Any cause of a low oxygen content in the blood may cause breathlessness and tiredness. There are several reasons including the following:

1. A low haemoglobin level: this is called anaemia. Haemoglobin is the protein in the red cells which carries the oxygen around the body. If a person is anaemic, there is less haemoglobin to carry the oxygen. The haemoglobin level may be low for several reasons. Anaemia may result from blood and iron loss due to heavy periods or bleeding from the gut. The haemoglobin may also be low if there is a low level of vitamins needed for its manufacture. These vitamins are folate and vitamin B_{12}. There are other less common causes of anaemia related to other diseases. Anaemia can make people feel tired, breathless, and weak. Occasionally, people who have normal heart arteries but who have severe

anaemia may get angina. This is not because blood cannot get to the heart muscle, but because the blood reaching the heart muscle does not contain enough oxygen. The blood, not the arteries, is the problem.

2. Damage to the lungs lowers the concentration of oxygen uptake in the blood:

    ◆ smoking-related lung disease (bronchitis and emphysema)

    ◆ blood clots in the lungs arteries (pulmonary emboli)

    ◆ lung scarring (lung fibrosis)

    ◆ serious lung infections (pneumonia)

    ◆ cancers destroying the lung tissue

    ◆ congestion of the lungs with water.

3. A lower concentration of oxygen at high altitude (e.g. in Peru or at the top of a mountain).

4. Holes in the heart: the right and left heart should be completely separated by partition walls called the interartrial and interventricular septums. Some babies are born with a hole in the septum and so blood can flow from the one side to the other. After a while, blood may flow from the right to the left side of the heart without going to the lungs. The babies have a low concentration of oxygen in their blood because the blood has not flowed through the lungs to pick up oxygen. They are called 'blue babies' because their lips and tongue look blue due to the reduced level of oxygen in their blood. The treatment is to diagnose the condition as soon as possible and to seal up the hole. In some cases this is done while the fetus is still in the womb, but in most cases it is done after birth.

Fuel and oxygen for the organs

The cells making up every part of our body—the brain, skin, bones, arms and legs, muscles, liver, kidneys, gut, and every other organ—need fuel and oxygen to perform their functions. Without sufficient oxygen, the cells die. For example, if a heart artery supplying the heart muscle with blood and nutrients is blocked, the heart muscle cells die. This is a heart attack and can be fatal. The same applies to the brain when a person has a stroke. Some organs, like the liver and skin, may be damaged but they have good repair mechanisms. Others, like the brain, do not recover as well.

The circulation of blood to the lungs

The large lung (pulmonary) arteries are like the large water pipes coming from a reservoir to supply an entire town. These are big enough to cope with surges in demand from all areas of the town at the same time. These large lung vessels give rise to several other large pipes which supply sections of the town. These give rise to medium-sized pipes supplying single streets. Smaller pipes supply individual houses. Within each house there are many even smaller pipes which supply individual taps and appliances.

Large pulmonary arteries supply whole lungs or whole sections of lung. These large vessels can cope with huge changes in demand. There are large changes in the volume and flow of blood through the lungs depending on what we are doing. When we sleep or rest, the blood flow around the body and the lungs is relatively small. When we run or do vigorous exercise, the blood flow and volume increases sharply to five times the sleeping flow rate and volume.

Medium-sized pulmonary arteries control flow to a single small segment of the lung. If this area of the lung is temporarily not getting air for some reason, perhaps because the person has pneumonia, these lung arteries must be able to actively shut down supply, so as not to waste blood and energy. However, they must be also able to increase flow to this segment of lung as demand for blood increases when the pneumonia has resolved.

Such fine control of blood flow to areas of the lung is an active process. The medium-sized lung arteries have 'muscular' walls which can widen or narrow down. This allows fine tuning and precise control of the blood supply to an area of lung depending on local demand.

Exercise, the circulation, and the lungs

During exercise the arm and leg muscles need more fuel. The heart has to pump more blood, nutrients, and oxygen around the body so that the muscles can do their work.

This increased demand for blood by the muscles has to be met by an increase in supply from the heart. This depends on both sides of the heart being able to pump an increased amount of blood when necessary. The lungs also have to be functioning normally so that oxygen can get into the blood. Normal lung arteries can cope with the increased blood flow by becoming wider. In PAH, the lung arteries are thickened and narrow and cannot expand, and so the blood flow around the circulation is restricted. This results in a lower oxygen level in the blood, so that PAH patients are breathless when they exercise.

The main way that the heart pumps more blood around the circulation is by pumping faster. That is why we feel or hear our heartbeat when we exercise. The faster the heart rate, the more blood is pumped around the circulation. Marathon runners and other athletes, who exercise to very high levels and train almost every day, often have a slow heart rate. This is because their heart is thickened and larger and beats more efficiently. A person who does little or no exercise may have a heart rate at rest of 70 bpm (beats per minute). A trained athlete's heart rate (pulse rate) may be as slow as 50 bpm (or lower with endurance training). Their heart can deliver a similar amount of blood but at a slower heart rate. When athletes exercise or run, their heart rate may increase to only 90 bpm, whereas an untrained person's heart rate may be considerably faster.

Training improves the efficiency of the heart, the lungs, the circulation, and the ability of the arm and leg muscles to extract oxygen from the blood. This is why when we become fitter, we feel generally better and more able to do things.

Exercise for patients with PAH

Most patients with PAH should exercise. They should exercise to reasonable, sensible levels but not overdo things. They should stop if they feel light-headed, faint, or very breathless.

4

Blood pressure

 Key points

- Blood pressure is the pressure in the arteries.
- Normally, in adults of all ages, the pressure should be at or below 140/85 mmHg.
- If the blood pressure is too high for long periods of time, there may be damage to the inside wall of the arteries in the brain, neck, eye, heart, and kidneys, the aorta, and the leg arteries.
- High blood pressure increases the risk of stroke and heart attack.

What is blood pressure?

Blood could not move and circulate around the body unless it was pumped by the heart. Without pressure pushing blood around the arteries, blood would stay still, like water in a garden hose with the tap turned off.

The pressure in the arteries depends on the following:

- The power of the heart pump: if the pump is weak, the pressure may be low.
- The volume of blood in the circulation: if there is little blood in the circulation, for example after a large loss of blood, the pressure may be low.
- The resistance against which the heart has to pump: this depends on the diameter of the smaller arteries called arterioles. Arterioles are medium-sized blood vessels with muscular walls. The blood pressure is mainly controlled by narrowing and widening of the walls of arterioles. Their diameter is controlled by nerves and chemicals secreted by our glands (adrenaline and noradrenaline—the 'fight or flight' substances). When the arterioles are narrowed, the resistance to blood flow is high and the blood pressure is high. If the arterioles are relaxed and wide open, the resistance to blood flow is low and the pressure is low.

What is systemic or the common type of hypertension?

The common type of hypertension, a high blood pressure in the main arteries, is sometimes called *systemic* hypertension. Systemic refers to the systemic blood circulation and not the pulmonary (lung) circulation. This is to distinguish it from PAH.

Why is blood pressure recorded with two numbers, one on top of the other?

The number on top is the pressure in the arteries when the heart is contracting, pushing blood around the systemic circulation. This is the **systolic** phase of the cardiac cycle. This upper number is called the systolic level of a person's blood pressure.

The lower number is the pressure in the arteries when the heart is relaxing and filling with blood. This takes place during the **diastolic** phase of the cycle and is called the diastolic blood pressure.

A pressure of 120/80 mmHg means that if a tube containing the liquid metal, mercury, were attached to the artery, the column of mercury would rise to a height of 120 mm (12 cm). These experiments were carried out in horses many years ago and led to our understanding of the circulation.

Although we still record blood pressure in mmHg (millimetres of mercury), the traditional mercury blood pressure machines (sphygmomanometers) have been phased out because of the cost and difficulty in obtaining mercury, and also because mercury is poisonous. We now use automatic battery-powered digital machines. Patients can now record and monitor their blood pressure with these widely available and generally accurate machines.

All adults should have their blood pressure measured at least once every 5 years, or more if there is a question that they have a high blood pressure. This can be done by your GP.

Which number is more important?

Both figures are equally important.

The systolic recording is more commonly high in elderly people who have stiff non-elastic arteries. The surge of blood being ejected out of the heart is recorded as a higher number than normal because the walls of the arteries have lost their elasticity and ability to 'cushion' the sudden increase in pressure.

The diastolic recording is usually high in young people who have elastic arteries, but the overall tone of their arteries is high because they are narrow. Young people with high blood pressure typically have a normal systolic recording but a high diastolic recording.

What is a normal blood pressure?

Normal pressure is at or below 140/85 mmHg. Blood pressure changes from minute to minute depending on what we are doing or thinking about.

It is important to remember that in the same way as the heart rate speeds up and slows down from minute to minute, depending on what we are doing or thinking about, so does the blood pressure. This is why it can be misleading for blood pressure to be measured when people are stressed, tired, worried or have just stopped exercising. GPs and nurses are trained to measure a person's resting blood pressure after the person has been sitting quietly for at least 3 minutes.

It is common and expected for the heart rate to be faster than normal and for the blood pressure to be higher than normal when it is being checked in the GP's surgery or in hospital. This is called 'white coat syndrome'; it is very common and is due to stress. 'White coat syndrome' can be distinguished from sustained or permanent blood pressure by recording the blood pressure over a 24-hour period using a cuff and a special computerized recording machine worn around the waist. The cuff inflates automatically every half-an-hour or so during the day and night. A person whose blood pressure is normal most of the time does not need treatment. However, if the blood pressure is high most of the time, they would benefit from treatment.

What is high blood pressure?

High blood pressure is a level that is consistently higher than 140/85 mmHg during both day and night in a person of any age over a period of months. A level higher than this increases the risk of stroke, heart attack, and arterial problems. The high pressure in the arteries increases the stress on the inside of the arterial wall (Figure 4.1). The force from a high power jet spray cleaner is very much greater than the gentle flow of water from a garden hose on a concrete terrace. The high pressure damages the lining cells of arteries. Fat (cholesterol) is more likely to get deposited in the walls of arteries if the pressure is high.

Blood pressure is the measurement
of force applied to artery walls

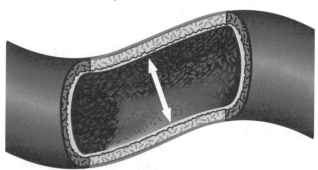

Figure 4.1 Blood pressure is the internal force driving blood through arteries. If the pressure is too high, the force damages the cells lining the internal wall of the arteries.

Only if the blood pressure is very high indeed, high enough to cause swelling of the brain, would a person have symptoms of hypertension. Almost always, hypertension is a silent disease. People with hypertension do not know they have it until their blood pressure has been measured. Therefore, high blood pressure has to be looked out for so that it can be found and treated before it is too late.

Hypertension is not treated like an infection with a course of treatment for a limited amount of time. Lifelong treatment is necessary. Once a patient starts treatment, they should continue it for life with regular checks of their blood pressure. More often than not, they will need increases in the amount of medication they take. Most people need two or more different types of blood pressure tablet. This is because the degree of hypertension tends to increase as we get older and it becomes more difficult to control.

 Fortunately, we have very good, safe, and effective tablets for treating hypertension, and most patients can be treated without encountering side-effects. Unfortunately, the tablets we use for systemic hypertension are of no use in treating PAH.

But doesn't the blood pressure depend on age?

Yes, but the pressure should be at or below 140/85 mmHg in an adult of any age, even the elderly. Doctors no longer 'allow' elderly patients to have a high blood pressure. Lowering a high blood pressure in an elderly person has similar benefits to lowering it in young adult.

If blood pressure is high, does a person always need tablets?

Yes. However, if a person is very fat, has a bad high-fat high-salt diet, and does no exercise, these 'lifestyle' factors can and should be reversed. Very often, particularly in young adults, when these risk factors are corrected and the person loses weight, exercises daily and has a healthy low-fat low-salt diet, their blood pressure comes down to normal and they can avoid tablets. Even if it does not come down completely to normal, it decreases to a level which requires lower doses of tablets and fewer tablets.

Treatment for hypertension is for life and should not be started until both the doctor and the patient are completely sure that the patient has hypertension.

Can high systemic blood pressure cause PAH?

No. But the high pressure in the body's arteries can put a strain on the left heart pumping chamber. This damages the heart muscle and causes a high pressure in the pumping chamber. This high pressure is transmitted back to the lung capillaries and to the pulmonary arteries. We call this post-capillary pulmonary hypertension. This means that the pressure in the lung arteries is high but not, as in PAH, because there is thickening or a problem in the lung arteries. The problem in *post-capillary pulmonary hypertension* is in the left side of the heart *after* or beyond or downstream from the lung capillaries (the word 'post' in medicine means *after*).

What is low blood pressure?

This is a pressure that is so low that the brain and kidneys are starved of blood and oxygen. Except when a person is acutely unwell, such as after substantial blood loss, this is very rare. As long as a person can think and can stand up without blacking out, and as long as the kidneys are working and getting enough blood, a low blood pressure is not important. Indeed, it is generally safer and better to have a pressure of 100/70 mmHg than 150/90 mmHg. A pressure below 100/60 mmHg could be considered 'low'.

It is quite common for people with normal blood pressure to feel faint or light-headed occasionally if they get out of bed quickly or stand up from a sitting position. This is because most of the blood is in the legs. Standing up lowers the blood pressure in the head and that is why we can feel light-headed if we stand up quickly. This is more common in people who are being effectively treated for high blood pressure with tablets. It may sound strange, but this is not a bad thing and suggests that the blood pressure is usually nice and low and well controlled. It is generally better for the blood pressure to be slightly low than to be high.

What problems occur with high blood pressure?

Figure 4.2 shows the main complications of persistent high blood pressure.

Brain

- ◆ Stroke.
- ◆ Dementia due to small strokes and damage to the brain.
- ◆ Headache only if the blood pressure is very high.

Eye

- ◆ Damage to the lining cells at the back of the eye (retina).

Neck

- ◆ Fat can form on the inside of the neck arteries. This can crack and bits of fatty material can travel in the blood to the brain causing strokes or short-lasting 'mini-strokes' (transient ischaemic attacks (TIAs)).

Heart

- ◆ Furring up and blockages in the heart arteries causing angina and heart attack.
- ◆ Thickening and weakening of the left heart muscle pump causing heart failure.

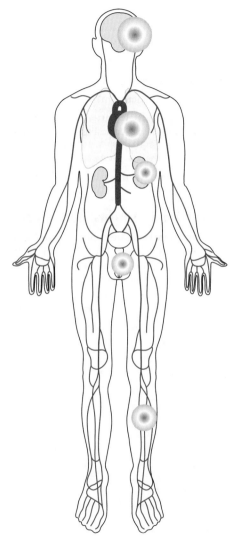

Figure 4.2 Sites in the body affected by high systemic blood pressure:

The high blood pressure damages arteries directly by high pressure and stress on the inside walls as well as increasing the risk of cholesterol deposits inside the arteries.

The eyes—causing damage to the retina and blindness; the heart arteries—causing heart attacks; the heart muscle—causing heart failure; the aorta—causing widening and weakening and aortic rupture; the kidneys—causing kidney damage and failure; the arteries to the penis—causing erectile dysfunction (impotence); the arteries to the legs—causing impaired blood supply (claudication).

Kidneys

◆ Kidney failure.

Aorta

◆ Tearing (dissection) of the aorta.

◆ Blow-outs in the aorta (aortic aneurysm).

◆ Furring up and blockages in the leg arteries (peripheral vascular disease) causing pain in the calf muscles when walking (claudication).

Penis

◆ Damage to the blood supply to the nerves of the penis causing erectile dysfunction.

Is systemic hypertension more common in PAH?

No. Systemic hypertension and PAH are completely different. However, long-standing inadequately controlled systemic hypertension can lead to a high pressure in the left ventricle. This high pressure is transmitted back through the lungs to the pulmonary arteries. This condition is called pulmonary hypertension (not pulmonary *arterial* hypertension, because the source of the problem is in the left heart and not the pulmonary arteries). The treatment of this sort of pulmonary hypertension is very different from treating PAH.

5

Palpitation

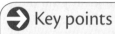
What is palpitation?

Palpitation is a symptom when a person feels their heartbeat or is aware of their heart.

Palpitation is often more noticeable when lying on the left side in bed. This is because the heart falls against the chest wall when lying on the left and vibrates against the inside of the chest. Some people can also hear their heart beat at night and might feel the heart beat pulsing in their neck or head. This is not serious as long as the heart rhythm is normal.

What are the causes of palpitation?

Palpitation can be due to a normal heart rhythm but the heart beat may be more forceful or faster than normal. Exercise and stress are common causes.

Palpitation may also be due to extra beats or abnormal heart rhythms. Extra beats are usually harmless. Occasionally, and more commonly in elderly people, palpitation can be due to an irregular rhythm in the collecting chambers. This is called atrial fibrillation.

There are several different types of abnormal heart rhythm. The seriousness of an abnormal heart rhythm depends largely on the state of the heart and its blood supply. If the heart muscle and its blood supply are normal, most heart rhythms are harmless. Patients with unpleasant palpitation should see their GP who may refer them to a heart specialist.

Finding the cause of palpitation

The only way a doctor can tell the cause of palpitation is by recording the heart rhythm with an electrical recording of the heart (electrocardiogram (ECG)) while the patient is experiencing the palpitation.

But the palpitation may last only a few seconds?

In that case, your doctor may advise you to have a 24 or 48 hour ECG recorder fitted so that your heart rhythm can be recorded and then analysed. But here again, some people have very intermittent palpitations. If they are intermittent and do not cause any symptoms of giddiness, blackouts, or chest pain, they are probably harmless and nothing to worry about.

Occasionally, people lose consciousness for a few seconds. This is frightening and should always be taken seriously and investigated. There are several causes, and occasionally no cause can be found. The problem is either in the head (brain problems) or in the heart (very slow or very fast heart rates and abnormal rhythms).

Is palpitation like a heart attack?

No. Palpitation is very different to a heart attack, which is due to blockage of a heart artery. This causes chest heaviness or arm tightness and breathlessness, and sometimes loss of consciousness. Palpitation is only occasionally due to a sudden lack of blood supply to the heart.

Heart attacks are very unusual in PAH unless the patient also has conditions which make cholesterol deposits in the arteries more likely. These are called risk factors. They are:

- smoking
- a high cholesterol level
- being overweight or obese
- diabetic
- systemic hypertension
- being fat or overweight
- taking little exercise.

Do palpitations need treatment?

It depends on the cause. Tablets to treat heart rhythm problems are usually quite effective, but occasionally can make the palpitation and the rhythm abnormality worse and reduce the power of the heart. Sometimes, special procedures (ablations) are done to treat abnormal heart rhythms.

Is palpitation common in PAH?

No. Patients with severe PAH may have a fast heart rate. A fast heart rate is faster than 100 bpm. This is because their heart has to work harder to pump blood around the circulation. The heart is beating faster because the right heart has to work harder to pump blood against a high pressure, and the right heart pump is weaker and so has to beat faster in order to supply blood and oxygen around the body. A few patients with PAH may have a fast heart rate due to an abnormal heart rhythm (arrhythmia). This is unusual. The two most common abnormal heart rhythms are atrial fibrillation and supraventricular tachycardia.

- Atrial fibrillation is a completely irregular rhythm originating in the collecting chambers.

- Supraventricular tachycardia is a fast regular rhythm due to abnormal electrical circuits between the collecting and pumping chambers.

6

What is PAH?

> ## ➜ Key points
>
> ◆ PAH is a high pressure in the *lung* arteries.
>
> ◆ PAH is very rare and more serious than 'ordinary' common hypertension, which is a high blood pressure in the *main* arteries.
>
> ◆ PAH can occur on its own or is associated with a several other conditions.
>
> ◆ The precise cause of PAH is unclear.
>
> ◆ Some forms of PAH occur in families and are due to a genetic problem.
>
> ◆ PAH results from defects in the cells of the lung arteries.
>
> ◆ Several new drugs are being used to try to correct these faults.

What is PAH?

The normal mean blood pressure (two-thirds of the difference between the systolic and diastolic pressure added to the diastolic pressure) in the lung arteries is around 15 mmHg.

In PAH, the mean pressure in the lung arteries is 25 mmHg or higher. Doctors often abbreviate the mean pressure recording in letters or reports to mPAP.

PAH is defined as a high pressure in the lung arteries without any other problem in the heart or lungs causing or contributing to the high pressure. The pump function of the heart (the output of blood ejected from the heart) is usually either normal or reduced.

PAH is rare

Whereas one person in 20 has coronary heart disease (blocked or narrowed heart arteries), only one person in 50 000 (that's only one person in a large town) has PAH. Therefore, compared with coronary heart disease or 'ordinary' hypertension, PAH is very rare. Having PAH is a bit like being struck by lightning—very unlikely to happen, but once it has happened the fact that it is rare is of no consolation to the patient.

What is the main problem in PAH?

The walls of the lung arteries become thicker and this causes narrowing of the artery. As the arteries become narrower, less blood flows through them.

The three main problems causing narrowed and, in some cases, blocked lung arteries are as follows.

◆ The artery walls become thicker.

◆ The arteries go into spasm and clamp down. This is because the walls of the arteries contain muscle fibres which can contract.

◆ Clots form inside the arteries.

What causes PAH?

In common with many other rare medical conditions, we don't know the precise cause of PAH. We are, however, making a lot of progress. Scientists have identified several defects in some of the molecules and cells of the lung arteries. Some people have a certain gene, which makes them vulnerable to PAH. PAH is also associated with (linked to) other rare medical conditions.

A substance, which could be a protein or another type of molecule, sticks onto the surface of a lung artery cell. This is called a receptor. It's a bit like a docking station or mooring post. The protein and the receptor fit together like the two bits of a seatbelt. Once the protein is attached to the receptor, it can act as a signalling system to other molecules within the cell. Signals are sent by linked

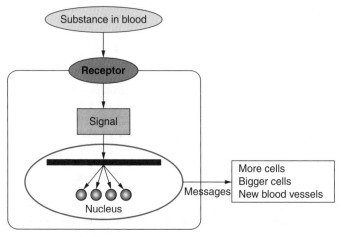

Figure 6.1 How PAH develops.

molecules, via many complex pathways, to the nucleus of the cell (Figure 6.1). The genes controlling the cell are located in the nucleus, a bit like a central computer in a large network. The genes send out messages to all the lung artery cells.

Several things can happen as a result of the faulty signal from the genes. The genes turn on all sorts of cell processes which are inappropriate for the needs of the cell. They turn a normal cell into a corrupt cell. It's a bit like Chinese whispers: the final message from the nucleus to the cells is garbled and completely wrong. In PAH, this incorrect message has serious implications.

Cell changes in PAH

With wrong signals being sent out to other lung artery muscle cells, previously normal cells in the wall of the lung artery multiply they become larger than they should be and move to places where they should not be. The filler material between the cells also becomes larger and new blood vessels form.

The inside of the artery virtually closes off, restricting blood flow. The muscular walls of the artery clamp down, further restricting blood flow through the artery. Blood clots form inside and these can block of the blood flow completely.

How do some of the drugs used to treat PAH work?

These drugs block the attachment of the substance in the blood to the surface of the lung smooth muscle cell. An example is endothelin receptor blockers (ERAs). These are commonly used to treat PAH.

The importance of the endothelial cells in PAH

The inner lining cells of the lung arteries are called endothelial cells. They form the inner lining of all vessels in the circulation, from the heart to the smallest capillary. The endothelial cells are very important in the control of the width of the blood vessel. The endothelium makes several substances—some open up the arteries and others close them down.

Nitric oxide

The endothelial cells produce a gas called nitric oxide (this is not the same as laughing gas, *nitrous* oxide) which widens arteries and keeps them open. This is called vasodilation and nitric oxide is called a vasodilator. It lasts in the blood for only a few seconds before it is changed to an inactive substance by a chemical called phosphodiesterase-5. Phosphodiesterase-5 is an important chemical because one of the types of drugs we use targets and blocks it. The drug is a phosphodiesterase-5 inhibitor. One of the types we use is called sildenafil (or Viagra) and another is called tadalafil (or Cialis). Both drugs are better known for the treatment of erectile dysfunction or impotence. These drugs do not cause erections when used to treat PAH. The destruction of phosphodiesterase-5 increases the level and duration of nitric oxide activity in the artery.

Endothelin

Endothelins are proteins produced by the endothelial cells. Endothelin is a very powerful constrictor of lung smooth muscle cells and blood vessels. It also causes scarring or fibrosis, growth of cells and inflammation. All these processes cause thickening of the lung arteries. Endothelin increases blood pressure. There are high levels of endothelin in patients with PAH.

One of the types of drugs we use to treat PAH prevents the endothelin attaching to the receptor on the surface of the lung smooth muscle cell. If endothelin cannot attach to the receptor, it cannot produce its dangerous effects in PAH.

Prostacyclin

Prostacyclin is a chemical which opens arteries. There are low levels of prostacyclin in the lung artery cells of patients with PAH. We treat PAH with prostacyclin-like drugs to open up the narrowed lung arteries.

Genetic causes of PAH

The genetic defect causing familial PAH has been identified. Several genetic defects (gene mutations) have also been found in 10% of patients with the type of PAH labelled as idiopathic (no known cause found).

PAH associated with connective tissue disease

This is quite a major and important type of PAH. By far the most common type of connective tissue disease associated with PAH is systemic sclerosis or scleroderma. Twelve per cent of patients with systemic sclerosis develop PAH. Patients with systemic sclerosis may also develop thickening and stiffness of the heart muscle, and this makes them breathless and tired.

Patients with systemic sclerosis may also have lung fibrosis, and occasionally kidney problems, in addition to the other characteristic problems of thickening of the skin—cold hands (Raynaud's disease), and gullet (oesophagus) and bowel problems.

We advise our rheumatology colleagues to screen patients with systemic sclerosis annually for PAH. Patients should be asked about breathlessness or tiredness; have a clinical examination, looking for signs of PAH; have a 6 minute walk test; a lung function test (breathing test); and an echocardiogram (heart ultrasound) to estimate the pressure in the lung arteries.

PAH also occurs in other connective tissue diseases, but less commonly than in systemic sclerosis. Patients with lupus, mixed connectival tissue disease, rheumatoid arthritis, dermatomyositis, and Sjögren's syndrome should be investigated for PAH if they feel breathless or tired.

Other conditions in which PAH might occur

PAH is associated with severe liver disease (cirrhosis), and human immunodeficiency virus (HIV) infection and haemolyte anaemia (fragile red blood cells). If there is any suggestion that PAH has occurred, the patient should be referred to a PAH centre for consideration for right heart catheterization to confirm or exclude the diagnosis, but how these conditions cause PAH is not known. PAH has also occurred in people taking the slimming drugs fenfluramine and dexfenfluramine (appetite suppressants) but these are no longer used.

Congenital heart disease

PAH occurs in people who were born with heart defects causing an increase in the flow of blood from the left side of the heart to the right. Adults born with congenital heart disease are now seen in special clinics called GUCH (grown-up congenital heart disease) clinics by specially trained cardiologists.

7

The difference between PH and PAH

→ Key points

- Pulmonary hypertension (PH) is a high pressure in the lungs.
- There are many causes of PH.
- PAH is a cause of PH due to a specific problem with the lung artery wall.
- The problem with PAH occurs before (pre) the lung arteries form capillaries. This is called 'pre-capillary PAH'.
- Pre-capillary PAH can be due to PAH, lung diseases, or clots in the lung arteries.
- Clinicians often talk about PH when strictly speaking they mean PAH.
- PH can be due to several problems with the left side of the heart, congenital heart problems, damage to the lungs due to smoking, clots in the lungs, and several other conditions.
- PH and PAH can be identified and distinguished using simple tests.

The difference between PH and PAH

In both conditions, the mean pressure in the pulmonary arteries is 25 mmHg or more.

Pre-capillary PH

Pre-capillary PH means that the cause of the high pressure is in the lung arteries, *before* (pre) the capillaries. The pressure in the left heart is normal (*at or below* 15 mmHg)

There are three main causes of *pre*-capillary PH:

1. An abnormality in the *walls of the lung arteries* (PAH).
2. *Lung problems* damaging or destroying the lung tissue thereby increasing the pressure in the lung arteries.

3. *Clots in the lung arteries* reducing the capacity for the lung arteries to carry blood. This causes an increase in the lung artery pressure.

Post-capillary PH

Post-capillary PH means that the cause of the high pressure in the lung arteries is *after* or *downstream* from the capillaries. This is diagnosed from the right heart catheter test which shows that the left heart pressure is high (*higher than* 15 mmHg).

There are several causes of post-capillary PH. Any condition resulting in weakness or a strain on the *left* pumping chamber can cause post-capillary PH by causing an increased back pressure through the pulmonary veins to the pulmonary arteries. Common examples are as follows:

1. Heart attacks or furring up of the heart arteries (coronary heart disease).

2. Systemic hypertension (ordinary hypertension).

3. Aortic or mitral valve problems:

   ◆ if the outflow or *aortic* valve is leaky or narrowed, the pressure in the left pumping chamber increases and this is transmitted back through the left collecting chamber to the lung arteries.

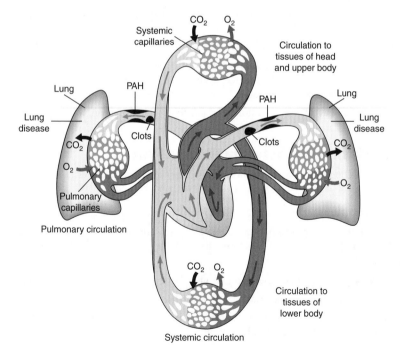

Figure 7.1 Pre-capillary and post-capillary pulmonary hypertension.

 ◆ if the inflow or *mitral* valve is leaky or narrowed, this increases the pressure in the left collecting chamber and this increased pressure is transmitted back through to the lung arteries.

4. Stiff heart or diastolic heart failure: here, the left heart does not relax normally. This condition is common in the elderly, the obese, and diabetics. Systemic sclerosis can also result in a stiff heart.

Classifying (pigeon-holing) the different types of PAH

The more we find out about medical conditions and what causes them, the easier it is to treat them. This is really important in PAH. The treatments we use in PAH depend on the type of PAH and its cause. Types of PAH caused by a similar mechanism are put in the same 'pigeon-hole' or classification.

PAH is due to abnormal growth and increased numbers of cells in the wall of the lung arteries, causing thickening and narrowing, with spasm of the arteries and a tendency to formation of blood clots in the arteries. We also understand some of the molecular and cellular abnormalities causing these changes.

Although we do not know the precise cause of PAH, we believe that *all* the types we have identified so far share similar features. When we look under a microscope at small bits of the arteries of patients who have different types of PAH, the arteries look similar. Different types of PAH also share similar molecular and cellular abnormalities. This means that whatever the type of PAH, the mechanisms causing it are the same. Therefore we can group all the different types of PAH into the same pigeon hole or classification. That is why we use the same forms of treatments for all of them.

Therefore, tailoring treatments to patients based on our understanding of the causes of the condition makes sense.

There are five main groups of conditions causing PH

1. PAH

2. PH due to heart problems (see above)

3. PH due to lung problems:
   ◆ smoking-related bronchitis and/or emphysema
   ◆ interstitial lung disease (fibrosis)
   ◆ sleep apnoea
   ◆ living at high altitude.

4. PH due to clots in the lungs

5. Miscellaneous causes and conditions with many different mechanisms are grouped together. There are many causes including:

    ◆ blood conditions: myeloproliferative disorders, splenectomy

    ◆ sarcoidosis, vasculitis

    ◆ Gaucher's disease, thyroid disorders

    ◆ chronic renal failure on dialysis.

Different types of PAH

Currently we group the different types of PAH as follows and treat all in a similar way.

1. Idiopathic (PAH of unknown cause, occurring on its own—the most common type).

2. Inherited: faulty genes have been identified (this type of PAH runs in families and is sometimes called familial).

3. Drugs: dieting drugs (fenfluramine is no longer used).

4. Conditions in which PAH occurs:

    ◆ connective tissue disease (systemic sclerosis or scleroderma is the most common)

    ◆ HIV infection

    ◆ long-standing liver problems (portal hypertension)

    ◆ congenital heart disease

    ◆ certain forms of anaemia (sickle cell disease).

PAH caused by congenital heart disease

PAH occurs in patients born with heart defects and blood flows from the left side to the right side of the heart. The abnormal connection between the left and the right side of the heart is called a shunt. PAH occurs because the pressure in the lung arteries increases due to increased volume and flow of blood.

Eisenmenger's syndrome

When the pressure in the lung arteries and the resistance to blood flow increases above the pressures in the left side of the heart, blood flows from the right to the left heart (Figure 7.2). Deoxygenated blood from the body returning to the right heart does not travel to the lungs for oxygenation. Instead, it flows directly from the right heart to the left heart. This is called Eisenmenger's syndrome. Patients with Eisenmenger's syndrome have blue tongues and lips and an increased number of red blood cells in an attempt to increase the oxygen-carrying capacity and oxygen concentration in their blood. Patients with Eisenmenger's syndrome are living longer now than they used to. Eisenmenger patients should

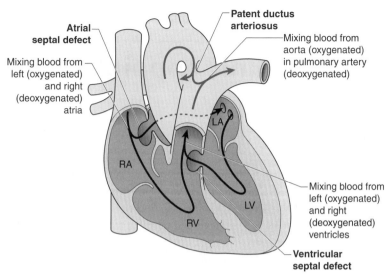

Figure 7.2 Connections between the left and right sides of the heart can result in pulmonary hypertension. Blood flows from the high pressure side to the low pressure side. Normally the pressure in the left or systemic circulation is higher than in the right or pulmonary circulation. If there is a significantly big hole in the heart with blood flowing from left to right through either a ventricular or atrial septal defect, the resistance to blood flow in the lung arteries increases. This results in a high pressure in the lungs – pulmonary hypertension. When the pressure in the right side of the heart is greater than in the left the blood flows from right to left. This means that blood is not getting to the lungs and the oxygen level of blood flowing around the body is low. This causes breathlessness, a blue tongue and lips (cyanosis) and other problems. This situation is called Eisenmenger's syndrome.

be advised of the risks of pregnancy and given advice about contraception. If pregnant, termination should be discussed. Once Eisenmenger's syndrome has occurred, it is too late to correct the fault.

There are some patients with a lesser degree of shunting because the pressure in their lung arteries is not so high. In these patients, blood may flow from both left to right and right to left.

8

Your clinic appointments

➔ Key points

- Your PAH clinic appointments are important for you and your family.
- The appointments allow you to ask your specialist team anything you want to know about your condition.
- Preparing for clinic appointments and travelling to and from clinic can be stressful and tiring.
- Write down any questions you may have.
- Bring your medications with you.
- Do not hesitate to phone after a clinic appointment if there is something you are not sure about or something that has confused you.

Specialist PAH clinics and outreach clinics

Each of the main PAH centres in the UK runs clinics in its own way, and there may be differences in the way that they are run. You may also be seen in an outreach clinic. This is in a hospital which is not one of the specialist PAH centres but is nearer to your home. The outreach clinic is run by a local consultant. One of the specialist consultants from a PAH centre also attends. The aim of outreach clinics is to make life easier for the patient. There is a shorter distance to travel and 'taking the specialist PAH centre to the patient' makes life quite a lot easier. Most patients prefer to see the PAH specialist with their local medical and nursing team at a local hospital.

Bring someone with you

It is sensible and practical to bring someone with you, at least for your first clinic appointment. This is helpful whatever your state of health. Your husband or wife, family member, or a close friend will take you to the clinic, help you carry any bags you may have (snack, book, medications), drive you to the clinic and park the car, or help you navigate public transport.

Hospital transport, however, may not allow you to travel with someone because there may not be enough room in the car and this is something you should find out from your PAH team when they make your appointment.

Perhaps most importantly, whoever accompanies you will remind you about what you were told in clinic. Most patients find it difficult to take in and remember everything they have been told by the doctors and nurses. If English is not your first language or you have hearing difficulties, it is really important to bring an interpreter or someone else with you to explain what is going on.

The main purpose of the clinic appointment

The main aim of the clinic is for the patient to be able to ask the clinician (and patients see both doctors and nurses) questions about their condition, to explain what tests they need and what is involved, and what changes need to be made to their medications. Blood tests, X-rays, scans, ECGs, breathing tests, and other tests may be done on the same day.

If you are worried about symptoms which you think may be due to your condition or your medications, there is no better place to discuss it than face to face with your clinical team. Telephone calls and the helpline are usually very reassuring for patients, but nothing beats a face-to-face consultation. The clinician can examine you, ask questions arising from your symptoms or the examination, and arrange tests which can be done while your are there. You can get the answer there and then and go home fully reassured.

In some centres, patients are admitted to hospital for tests or changes to their treatments. In most centres in the UK however, patients attend the PAH outpatient clinic and go home the same day.

Information from the clinic appointment and computer screen

We are all living in the computer world and this has generally greatly improved clinical care for patients. Assuming that the results of tests have been entered on the hospital database, all the results of your blood tests, scans, and other tests will be available at the click of a mouse. Clinical details of your history and examination, walking tests, heart ultrasound, catheter tests, and other information are also entered on to a database so that we have ready access to your clinical information.

The bad thing about computers in clinical care is that clinicians are forced to look at the screen rather than at the patient during the consultation. This is quite an important problem, and in recent years patients visiting their GP health centre or polyclinic, or a hospital clinic, have told us that these important consultations are more like an experience at an airport check-in desk than a very personal communication with their doctor. Unfortunately, this is 'progress' and it is the responsibility of doctors to make sure that they 'connect' with the patient and not only with the computer!

Furniture arrangements in clinic

The desk in the consulting room acts as a physical barrier which, unfortunately, may also impede and fog communication between the patient and the doctor. This can be solved if the doctor invites the patient to sit to the side of the desk rather than directly behind it. There should be room for at least one of your family or a friend to sit down with you. Patients in wheelchairs can also position themselves conveniently and comfortably.

Your test results belong to you

All the results from your tests belong to you, and you can always ask for copies of tests and copies of letters we send to your GP and other specialists involved in your care. In most hospitals, patients are copied in to the correspondence unless they do not want to be.

Preparing for your clinic appointment

This can be quite stressful, particularly for your first clinic appointment. Remember, the appointment is not an examination or test. It is an important and hopefully, pleasant educational and reassuring visit with your PAH team. They have only one interest—your welfare. They want to do everything they can to help you.

Before you come to clinic, make sure that you do the following:

◆ Write down any questions and ask them when you come. Bring a notebook and pen to make notes if you wish.

◆ Bring all your medications and tablets with you.

◆ If you have a rather complex health history, write down the conditions and dates when they occurred, and who treated them and at which hospital. This is useful because the clinician will be able to write to the other medical teams for more information about you if necessary.

◆ Make sure that you eat and drink before you start on your journey and bring a snack or some sandwiches and something to drink.

◆ Bring a book to read in case you have to wait at some stage on the journey or when you arrive in clinic. Most hospitals are very sensitive to patients' waiting times, but there are sometimes unavoidable delays due to all sorts of events out of the control of the PAH team.

◆ Hospital transport is a wonderful facility but does not always run to time. Please remember that the PAH team do all they can to make the journeys to and from hospital stress free, but this is not always possible.

◆ If you use oxygen, bring enough with you for the return journey.

◆ If you do not speak English, it is very important for you to bring an interpreter so that you can ask any questions you want and can understand the entire consultation. There are telephone interpreting services in the NHS and these are useful for patients who do not speak or understand English.

◆ Below, you will see the sort of questions you might be asked at any clinic appointment. Try to prepare the answers to these or jot down a few notes to help you when you come to clinic. The more we know about you and your condition, the easier it is for us to help you.

Your first visit

This can be very stressful indeed and we are sensitive to the way you feel. Meeting new doctors in a strange hospital, often in a crowded, uncomfortable, and busy clinic full of patients looking unwell, is certainly not a pleasant prospect. But it is necessary.

Leave plenty of time to get to hospital. However unpleasant, boring, and frustrating it is to have to wait to see the doctor and the PAH team, it is far less stressful than being late and possibly missing your appointment. Most PAH centres are very well run and organized, and patients are usually seen on time with minimal delays. Because in most countries there are only a few PAH centres serving the whole country, many patients live far from the PAH centre and may have to travel to the centre the day before their appointment.

We are looking forward to seeing you, meeting you and your family, and having the opportunity to getting to grips with your problem and sorting it out.

Subsequent visits

After your first visit you become one of the family! You will meet all the team, and get to know them more and more, as they will get to know you, with every visit. You will feel more comfortable and less stressed with every visit. It is important that you feel able to talk to all members of the team and understand them, and that they understand you. With time, you will be able to concentrate on yourself and how you are, rather than being apprehensive or anxious about the PAH team.

PAH team members and 'off days'

Like everyone, the members of the PAH team may have an 'off day'. There are many causes for this. Doctors and nurses work under considerable pressure and often administrative problems—lost notes, unavailable test results, late transport, waiting times for tests, hot and stuffy clinic areas—are out of their direct control. However, they are highly trained professionals, and are expected by everyone to be perfect, unhurried, unstressed, humorous, warm, and friendly to every patient every day. If you think that a PAH team member is 'off form' or having an 'off day', have some sympathy for them. They should have recovered by the time of your next clinic visit!

Test results and reports

We should have a letter from the specialist or doctor who referred you and copies of results of tests you have already had. These usually include a heart ultrasound and breathing tests which alerted the doctor that your symptoms could be due to PAH. The other tests you may have had are likely to be blood tests and a chest X-ray, and some referring specialists, particularly chest specialists, may have done scans of your lungs to look for clots or scarring.

Please give any other information, bags of tablets and medications, and details of previous illnesses and medical reports to the doctor. The more information we have about you, the better.

Do not be concerned or worried if the PAH specialist tells you that some tests may need to be repeated. This may be necessary in some patients to check borderline test results or some test results may not be available from the referral letter. The tests take a little time, but it is really important for us to have all the information we need to be able to tell you if you have PAH or not and if so, how severe it is and what treatment you should have. The test results may suggest that your symptoms may be due to some other medical condition and we may need to investigate this possibility.

The history

The importance of the history: narrowing down the possibilities

The doctor will want to know how you feel, when the symptoms started, and how they affect you. Very often we want to know when you were last '100% well'. Sometimes this can be quite difficult to answer, but it is really helpful to the medical team to understand when you first noticed even little things which you may have initially dismissed, but may have been the first manifestations or signs of your condition.

You will be invited to tell the history of your symptoms in your own time and in your own way, but the doctor may interrupt you from time to time to clarify a point. If you do not want to give the history yourself or cannot give the history for any reason, please ask a relative or friend to do this. There are some very important bits of the history that we need to know because the information affects the tests we arrange and the treatment we advise.

Talking to someone may not seem like much of a test, but in reality 80% of the information leading to a diagnosis is obtained in this way. To understand how powerful this is as a test, it is worth digressing and thinking about someone who finds that they can no longer walk to the local shops without stopping. We need to know why they have to stop, how long they have to stop for, and why precisely they have to stop. The problem could be a heart or lung or leg problem, or just old age and being fat or unfit, or, and this is very common in medicine, a combination of several things. The history can tell us. It is probably the most important part of medicine.

Perhaps the patient has to stop because they become breathless when walking. This could be a lung problem (bronchitis, emphysema, asthma, lung fibrosis, a chest infection or pneumonia, or lung cancer. Breathlessness can also be due to heart failure. Of course, it is the most common symptom in patients with PAH. However, as you can see, there are several other more common causes of breathlessness.

Alternatively, the patient may be experiencing chest tightness with or without some breathlessness. This could be due to angina. This is caused by furring up or blockages in the heart arteries.

Another possibility is that they may have to stop or slow down not because of breathlessness or chest discomfort, but because they experience cramp in the calves of their legs. We call this claudication. This is due to blockages or narrowing in the arteries of their legs. Most people with claudication have smoked.

Arthritis or muscle conditions also cause pain in the hips and knees, making it difficult for people to walk.

When did it start?

The symptom may have started:

- instantaneously, like sudden chest pain, suggesting a clot blocking a heart artery (heart attack)
- over seconds, like wheeziness due to obstruction of an airway (asthma)
- over days, suggesting infection (chest infection)
- over months suggesting degenerative conditions or tumours
- over a year or so, which is characteristic of PAH.

Any other symptoms or history of other medical conditions?

There may be other symptoms that point to the diagnosis such as a temperature suggesting infection, bleeding suggesting anaemia, or weight loss suggesting cancer. Finally, there may be background information which helps; for example, smoking (bronchitis, asthma, lung cancer), their parents died of heart attacks in their 40s (high cholesterol causing heart artery blockages and angina), or they have diabetes (furring up in the heart and leg arteries).

Pulmonary emboli (clots in the lungs)

Fairly sudden and severe breathlessness in a person who had been lying in bed after an operation, or has been on a lot of long-haul flights, or who has been immobilized with their leg in a cast for several weeks may be due to clots in the lung (pulmonary emboli). These are very serious and it is very important to confirm or exclude these urgently. Patients with suspected pulmonary emboli should be admitted to hospital for investigations (scans) and treated immediately with blood thinners (heparin) until the diagnosis of pulmonary emboli has been excluded by scans. If the scan shows clots in the lungs, warfarin is given for at least 6 months.

Patients with PAH are susceptible to pulmonary emboli. In some patients, pulmonary emboli are the cause of the PAH. In either case, PAH patients are treated 'lifelong' with warfarin.

Sudden left heart failure with fluid in the lungs

Sudden breathlessness and wheeziness when lying flat in bed, and increasing breathlessness when walking up hills, are characteristic of sudden left heart failure (left ventricular failure). Some people with left heart failure cough up pink frothy fluid. This is the water that has leaked from their lung capillaries into the air sacs of their lungs (alveoli) due to the effect of gravity when they lie in bed. This is a serious condition. A chest X-ray and heart ultrasound, and possibly a coronary angiogram (injecting contrast into the heart arteries), confirm the diagnosis and will point to the cause. A heart attack or long-standing heart failure are the most common causes. The condition can be controlled by water tablets (injections in the emergency situation) and other medications.

Chest infections and lung cancer

A smoker who has gradually become breathless over the past 3–5 years, and who presents with a temperature, cough, and severe breathlessness with wheezing, almost certainly has bronchitis. Weight loss and loss of appetite are very serious features in a smoker and suggest lung cancer.

 The history is extremely helpful. In many cases, it gives the doctor nearly all the information needed to diagnose the most likely cause of a patient's problem.

PAH

In PAH the most important symptom is breathlessness; this tends to develop slowly but progressively over a period of several months. Young children, who often do not recognize that they should stop when breathless but keep going until they black out, are an exception to this rule.

The typical PAH history is different from smokers' lung disease, which gradually worsens over many years and leads to attacks of bronchitis (producing breathlessness at rest when 'colds go to the chest'). PAH breathless is also different from heart failure, which may cause progressive breathlessness on exercise over months. It is associated with attacks of breathlessness at rest, for example when lying flat for prolonged periods (such as in bed at night).

Once PAH has become a serious consideration, we seek further clues from the history.

♦ Is there a family history of PAH or of unexplained deaths in young relatives?

♦ Occasionally, PAH is genetic. If so, it is important to examine other members of the family.

♦ Did you ever take slimming tablets? In the 1990s fenfluramine and dexfen-fluramine were promoted to help weight loss but were withdrawn after they were found to cause PAH and other problems. Please tell your PAH team about any tablets, even herbal ones, that you take or have taken over a period of time in the past. Although there is no evidence that non-prescription drugs cause PAH, discoveries are often made from similar findings in other patients, in the same way as we discovered the dangers of slimming tablets.

♦ Have you ever had clots in the legs or lungs? Pulmonary emboli cause breathlessness by blocking off the lung arteries and reducing blood flow to the lungs. However, pulmonary emboli can also cause PAH by a different mechanism.

♦ It is important to tell the PAH team *all* the medical conditions that you have had in the past. Things that you think are irrelevant may not be.

The history is so important that the same questions are often asked again and again—the same principle that is used by police to get confessions! This is partly due to inefficiency (junior staff followed by senior staff), but also because, after having been asked the questions, patients begin to mull over the story in their own mind and discuss their symptoms with their family. After thinking about their history, they remember things which they had previously thought were irrelevant, but to us are important and helpful.

Don't be put off or become irritated if we ask you similar questions about your history every time you come to clinic. It is not that we don't believe you or that we have forgotten what you said the last time. It is because we are interested in you and your history. Every PAH patient has a different history and is unique.

The heart in PAH: how bad are the symptoms?

The history also helps us get an idea of how the right heart is coping with the high pressure in the lungs. This is really important. We need to know how bad your symptoms are and how they affect your ability to walk, to work, to do housework, gardening, and shopping, and all other aspects of your daily life.

If the heart is coping perfectly, you will find that you are able to exercise normally, including running and walking long distances fast on the flat. When the heart is not normal but not seriously weakened, PAH patients can walk comfortably on the flat but find hills and stairs a problem and they become breathless after a flight of stairs. When the heart is significantly weakened, walking more that a few hundred metres on the flat becomes a struggle.

Breathlessness when washing, dressing, or talking on the telephone, or doing nothing, all indicate that the heart is severely weak. Feeling faint or actually losing consciousness on exertion, getting out of bed or out of a chair, are also serious symptoms which we need to know about.

Grading the severity of your symptoms

Our PAH patients are put into four classes depending on how severely they are affected. The grading system was devised by the World Health Organization and so you may see them referred to as WHO class or functional class—how well you 'function' and your ability to do things.

Class 1 No limitation in physical activity. Ordinary activities do not cause undue breathlessness or fatigue, or black-outs, or a feeling of light-headedness.

Class 2 Slight limitation of physical activities. These patients are comfortable at rest, but ordinary physical activities cause undue breathlessness, fatigue, chest pain, or faintness.

Class 3 Marked limitation of physical activities. These patients are comfortable at rest. Less than ordinary activities cause undue breathlessness, fatigue, chest pain, or faintness.

Class 4 Unable to carry out any physical activity without symptoms. These patients have signs of right heart failure, are often breathless at rest, and cannot speak for long on the telephone without becoming breathless.

Using the WHO classification to assess your response to treatment

The WHO categories influence the types of treatment we prescribe. They also tell us and other clinicians whether or not you are responding to treatments. We do not currently treat patients in class 1 with special 'disease-targeted therapies' because there is no good evidence at the moment that patients would benefit. This situation may change in the future.

At each visit, we ask how you are and what level of activities you can do before you get breathless. You may be asked: 'How far can you walk and how many steps or stairs can you climb before you get breathless and have to stop?' The reason we ask is simple. If you are finding things more difficult and are less able to walk and carry out normal daily activities, then we consider whether we should change your treatments.

Relationship of WHO class to test results

There is a rather loose relationship between WHO functional class and test results. Some people, particularly younger patients who have strong hearts, may remain quite fit and have only mild symptoms, but the echocardiogram and right heart catheter tests show a high pressure in their lungs.

The examination

The most important information obtained on examination in the setting of pulmonary hypertension is whether there is evidence of disease leading to pulmonary hypertension.

◆ We look at your *face and hands* carefully.

◆ We count the *pulse rate* at your wrist. This should be between 50 and 100 bpm. If it is higher than 100 bpm, this suggests one of several things: the patient is very nervous, has an overactive thyroid gland in the neck, has just rushed into the clinic and has not had enough time to relax before being examined, has recently taken a ventolin inhaler for asthma, or has a weakened heart due to PAH.

◆ We look and may press over your *feet and ankles* to see if there is excess fluid due to right heart failure.

◆ We look at the *venous pulsation in your neck* by asking you to rest your head against the pillow or head of the examination couch. The venous pressure is the height of the pulsation in the neck veins above the joint where the second rib is attached to the breast bone. The height of the venous pulse should be less than 6 cm. If the venous pulsation or pressure is higher than 10 cm, this indicates that the pressure in the right collecting chamber, into which the neck veins drain, is high. This is consistent with PAH causing weakness of the right heart.

◆ We feel the front of your chest to see if there is *abnormally strong pulsation* from your heart. Changes in the heart in response to high pressure only become obvious on examination very late. Either the heart can become very strong and muscular to deal with the high pressures, causing it to lift the chest slightly every time it beats, or it can become large and flabby, allowing fluid to collect in the ankles and neck veins. As always, it is never really either/or but a combination of both responses, with a bit of each happening at the same time. Because the changes on examination are very late or not specific enough (most ankle swelling has nothing to do with pulmonary hypertension), we need to diagnose pulmonary hypertension before there is much to find. This is where the tests we perform come in.

◆ We take the *blood pressure* from your arm or both arms and may check it a number of times. Patients who have long-standing high systemic pressure (ordinary blood pressure) may develop PH (as opposed to PAH). The distinction can be made at right heart catheterization.

◆ *Scleroderma or systemic sclerosis* is one of several connective tissue diseases which are associated with PAH. Systemic sclerosis causes (and literally means) *thickening of the skin especially on the fingers*, and *tightening of the skin around the nose and mouth*, and causes enlarged skin blood vessels on the face, called telangiectasia. Most patients also have gut problems with reflux and acid indigestion, and attacks of diarrhoea or constipation. Twelve per cent of patients with systemic sclerosis may develop PAH, but we do not know which patients do and which ones do not. Therefore we look carefully at your face and hands, and we ask you about your swallowing, indigestion, and bowel habits.

◆ Long-standing *liver disease* usually makes the liver large enough to feel, and causes pink discoloration of the palms. Some patients may be jaundiced, and the whites of their eyes look slightly yellow. Some patients have cirrhosis due to excess alcohol, but others may have caught an infection of the liver called hepatitis from blood transfusions or other causes.

◆ Severe *lung disease* usually leads to added sounds being heard when listening to the lungs during deep breathing. That is why we ask you to sit forward and take deep breaths in and out through your mouth. The crackles are due to fibrosis or scarring in the lungs. Lung fibrosis causes PAH, but PAH can also occur as a separate condition. Patients with smoking-related lung disease (bronchitis and emphysema) may have wheezes, and those with dominant emphysema (they usually occur together) have quiet breath sounds.

◆ Left heart disease is a weakness of the heart muscle caused by valve abnormalities, furring up and blockages of the heart arteries, and less commonly, certain heart muscle conditions. We listen for heart murmurs and other added sounds which point to the problem. Some adults are born with heart defects, for example holes in the heart or valve problems. Because of better medical care, they are living longer into adulthood. The increased flow of blood to the lungs can after several years lead to PAH.

Increased pressure in the lung arteries by itself causes no real changes on examination, unless it is very high indeed. In these severe cases, there may be an abnormal heart sound due to sudden closure of the valve regulating blood flow to the lungs from the right ventricle (the pulmonary valve).

What to do at when you are at home and are worried about something

Most UK PAH centres provide a telephone helpline during working hours. This is a very good and quick way to ask the specialist nurses any questions you may have about your condition or the treatments or other practical issues.

Common questions and concerns that patients have include symptoms they think might be due to medications, getting hold of medications, what to do if they forget to take a tablet or if they take too many tablets, having check blood tests for liver function if they are taking an endothelin receptor antagonist, practical arrangements for getting to clinic, problems with infusion pumps, oxygen supplies, dietary advice, whether they can drink alcohol or not, how much exercise they can do safely, and feelings of depression, fear, and insecurity.

Some women will want advice about contraception. Those who have been referred for surgery, removal of blood clots from the lung arteries, or lung transplantation, often have understandable anxieties about the wait to be seen in the surgical centre and other issues, which are generally best dealt with by the PAH team at the surgical centre although your 'home' PAH team will be able to give you advice.

9

Tests for PAH

➔ Key points

◆ Tests are necessary to see whether a person has or does not have PAH. Tests are also done to monitor patients and to see if they are responding to treatments.

◆ All the tests provide useful information. Each test result is like a piece of a jigsaw—the more pieces we have, the clearer and more complete the picture.

◆ The single most important test which either confirms or excludes PAH is a right heart catheter test. There is a small risk (1 in 1000) of death, arrhythmia, or lung or leg damage with this test.

◆ The other tests we do are either harmless or have a negligible risk.

◆ Blood tests can be done at your GP surgery. Other tests, including lung function, echocardiography (heart ultrasound), and lung scanning, may also be necessary and may be done at your local hospital.

Tests for breathless patients

There are many causes of breathlessness. By the time you have been referred to a PAH unit, you would have had quite a few tests, but we may need to repeat some of these or do other ones you have not had.

When a doctor sees a breathless patient for the first time, the common causes of breathlessness are considered first and then the less common ones. PAH is one of the least common causes of breathlessness.

PAH should be considered in patients with 'unexplained' breathlessness. 'Unexplained' means that the common causes have been excluded.

The common causes of breathlessness are:

◆ lung problems (smoking-related bronchitis, emphysema, asthma, lung fibrosis, lung cancer)

◆ heart problems (weak or stiff heart including coronary heart disease, faulty valves)

◆ low blood count (anaemia)

◆ being too fat

◆ being unfit.

PAH is not a common cause of breathlessness. But to you, it is the most important. It is also very important to us to make sure that we understand the causes of your symptoms and do everything we can to help you.

The following tests provide the information we need to diagnose PAH, assess its severity, and monitor patients who have PAH. We also do some of these tests in people who are susceptible to PAH, for example patients who have had clots in their lungs and those with systemic sclerosis (scleroderma), HIV, long-standing liver disease, or sickle cell anaemia.

Blood tests
What they tell us

We need to make sure that your breathlessness, fatigue and tiredness, or any other symptoms you may have are not due to a low blood count (anaemia), certain types of anaemia (sickle cell and thalassaemia can cause PAH), or a low thyroid level. We also need to make sure that your kidneys and liver (liver disease is another cause of PAH) are working normally, particularly if you are having treatments for PAH which can disturb the liver function in a small proportion of patients. HIV is a rare cause of PAH and so this blood test is important.

You may also have tests for your immune state to see if you have a connective tissue disease. These include scleroderma, lupus, rheumatoid arthritis, and Sjögren's syndrome. Each of these conditions may need treatment. You may already have been diagnosed with one of these conditions before you were referred to a PAH unit. If you have PAH and it is linked to another condition, we need to know about this, because treating the underlying condition often improves the PAH. A good example of this is lupus.

In advanced PAH, the right heart enlarges and the heart chambers stretch. This is because the heart has to work harder to pump blood into the narrowed lung arteries. A stretched heart produces high levels of a substance called brain natriuretic peptide (NT-proBNP or BNP) which is released into the blood. We measure this with the other blood tests we do to monitor your progress. The higher the level, the more the right heart is stretched, and this helps us to decide on the best treatment. Conversely, a low NT-proBNP suggests that the right heart is coping well, and this is good news.

What is involved?

Most people do not mind blood tests. If you think you might faint, tell the person taking your blood test. Ask if you can lie down on a couch while they take your blood. If there is no couch, sit back in a chair. A strap (tourniquet) will be tightened around your arm. Tell the person taking your blood which is the best vein for them to aim at! The needle does hurt a bit.

Make sure that the bleeding has stopped before you leave. It should take only a minute or two for the bleeding to stop, but may take longer in patients taking the blood thinner warfarin.

Chest X-ray

What it tells us

The chest X-ray shows the heart, lungs, ribs, and diaphragm. Solid tissues, like the heart and ribs, and solid areas in the lung appear white. Air looks black.

A chest X-ray is very helpful in people with lung symptoms (cough, phlegm, breathlessness, fever) who may have a serious chest infection (pneumonia), cancer, or lung fibrosis.

The chest X-ray is a simple and useful test for people who are breathless. A normal chest X-ray is reassuring and excludes serious pneumonia and other infections, lung fibrosis (scarring), cancer, lymphomas, and air in the pleural space (pneumothorax). With the development of newer and more accurate imaging techniques like high-resolution CT (HRCT) scans, the chest X-ray has become less important, but it remains a key test in a breathless patient.

Cancers or lymphomas are seen as white nodules or large solid areas, or spots in the ribs if the cancer has spread. We should emphasize that cancer is no more common in PAH than in people who do not have PAH. PAH patients are *not* at risk from cancer unless they have smoked.

The X-ray is not very helpful in confirming or excluding clots in the lungs unless these have resulted in severe PAH. If it is likely that you have had clots in the lung, you may be advised to have a perfusion lung scan, or a CT lung scan of your lung arteries (CTPA).

The lungs appear big and black on a chest X-ray in people who have smoked a lot. This is called emphysema. This is because the chemicals in tobacco destroy the lungs, which are replaced with air. Smokers are breathless because there is less lung tissue and fewer air sacs (alveoli) to transfer oxygen into the blood.

PAH occurs in 12% of patients with systemic sclerosis. Lung fibrosis (scarring) also occurs in some patients with systemic sclerosis. This makes the lungs look white and grainy. The more white and grainy the more widespread and severe is the fibrosis. Chest X-ray is also useful if heart disease is the cause of breathlessness, as it may show an enlarged heart and possibly fluid in the lungs.

In PAH without lung fibrosis or any other lung abnormality, the chest X-ray is of limited value and may be normal. In patients with severe PAH, the X-ray may show large lung arteries and a large heart resulting from the strain.

What is involved?

You have to remove your upper garments and stand next to an X-ray tube. A picture is taken while you take a deep breath in. The whole test takes only a minute or two. The radiation exposure is very small.

Most X-ray departments no longer produce large X-ray films that were stored in large envelopes. Gone are the days of doctors trying to find a recent X-ray from a large pile and then spilling all the X-rays on the clinic floor! Life has become simpler. Your X-ray will be uploaded onto the hospital computer system and we can look at your X-ray from a hospital computer.

Electrocardiogram (ECG)

What it tell us

An ECG is a tracing of the electrical activity of the heart. It shows the heart rhythm and rate. An ECG is very useful in patients who have had heart damage due to a heart attack. Heart attacks and coronary heart disease (furring up in the heart arteries) are *not* more common in patients with PAH.

The ECG shows several abnormalities in severe long-standing PAH. This is because the right heart gets larger and thicker because of the increased work it has to do. The changes are grouped together and referred to as right heart strain. They can be seen in about four out of five people with severe PAH. Some patients with severe PAH have abnormal heart rhythms and these can be identified on the ECG. These changes in a breathless patient may alert the doctor to request a heart ultrasound.

 A normal ECG does not exclude PAH.

What is involved

Sticky electrode pads are placed on the skin of the chest, arms, and legs while you lie on a couch. It is completely safe and painless, and takes less than a minute. The ECG is printed out on a piece of graph paper for you to take to your clinic appointment.

Echocardiography (heart ultrasound)
What is echocardiography?

> ❗ Echocardiography is the most important test for finding out why the heart might be the cause of breathlessness.
>
> ❗ All patients with suspected PAH should have an echocardiogram.

Echocardiography (*echo*, returning sound; *cardio*, heart; *graphy*, map of) is the same test as that used to take pictures of babies in the womb.

Echocardiography uses the same principle of physics that bats use to fly around. Bats cannot see well. They rely on echoes to find their way around deserted old buildings and derelict churches by making sounds which bounce off solid surfaces. The bats hear the echoes which tell them how far away they are from the roof and walls. Although the principle is the same, echocardiography is slightly more complicated than bat's echoes. The bat's echo system only needs to know how far away the wall is, not what the wall is made of and whether there are two walls with insulation between them.

When dealing with the heart, we need to know a lot more than how far away the heart is from the probe or transducer we put on the chest. We need to know the thickness of the heart walls, what the valves are like, the size of all four heart chambers, whether the heart is surrounded by fluid (which can occur if the heart is weak or inflamed), and how well the heart is working.

For these purposes, we use a very high frequency sound which is well above even the bat's hearing range. These high frequency sound waves don't just bounce off the chest wall or the surface of the heart. Most of the sound waves continue travelling on through all but the most solid structures. When the sound wave reaches a 'surface' (say the outside of the heart) most of the sound travels on but some echoes are sent back to the probe. The same happens when the sound reaches the inside of the heart where it meets blood, and so on. By some clever computer wizardry all the surfaces encountered can be reconstructed into a moving picture of the heart or a baby, depending on what you are looking at.

What it tells us

In the breathless patient, echocardiography tells us whether:

- the left heart and its valves are normal and working normally
- the right heart and its valves are normal and working normally
- there are any holes in the heart and the heart structure is normal
- it is likely or unlikely that the patient has PAH.

If the left heart is large and not working very well, we call this 'left heart failure'. This means that the muscle of the heart cannot do its work because the it has been weakened. Common causes of a weakened left heart are systemic high blood pressure, faulty heart valves, and coronary heart disease (furring up of the heart arteries) which reduces the blood supply to the heart and can also result in a heart attack with scarring of the heart muscle. The left heart also becomes stiff as we get older and does not relax normally. Weakness or stiffness of the left heart results in high pressure in the lungs. This is not PAH, which is due to a problem in the lung arteries themselves, but high back pressure from the left heart, which we call pulmonary hypertension (PH).

If the left heart is not working normally, we need to know the cause and what the best treatment is. We always try to find the cause and treat it. There are several good treatments (tablets and other forms of treatment) available which work for most people with ordinary (left) heart failure. If a valve is faulty, it may need replacement or repair.

Echocardiography and Doppler examination to measure the pressure in the lung arteries

The right heart is more difficult to see with echocardiography than the left heart because of its shape and position under the breast bone.

We measure the *ordinary (systemic) blood pressure* using a cuff wrapped around the upper arm and a blood pressure machine. To measure the *pressure in the lung arteries*, we use echocardiography and Doppler examination (named after Dr Doppler who discovered the Doppler effect on which the Doppler ultrasound technique is based). Doppler is part of the echocardiogram test. The principle of Doppler is similar to that used in police speed cameras. Speed cameras send out sound waves that bounce off your car. The frequency of the returning echo depends on how fast you are driving away from the speed camera.

In the heart, Doppler measures the speed of blood cells propelled by the heart as they move away from the probe on your chest. The higher the pressure in the blood vessel or heart chamber, the faster the blood cells move. Doppler is not very accurate, but it is more practical and much safer than sticking a tube inside the heart. The information we obtain from Doppler testing gives us a reasonable idea of the pressure in the lung arteries.

In PAH, the high pressure in the lung arteries is transmitted back to the right ventricle. The pressure in the right ventricle increases and this increases the back flow of blood from the right ventricle through the tricuspid valve to the right atrium (collecting chamber). The leak of blood from the right ventricle through the tricuspid valve (a minor leak of the tricuspid valave is normal) back into the right atrium can be detected and measured using Doppler scanning. The speed of blood (measured by Doppler) leaking back is used to estimate the pressure in the lung arteries.

- ◆ If the Doppler pressure in the lung arteries is low, this means PAH is unlikely.
- ◆ If the Doppler pressure in the lung arteries is very high, then it is very likely that the patient has PAH.
- ◆ However, the scan is inaccurate in borderline cases. Some results showing slightly high Doppler pressures will be normal when the pressure is measured by a catheter. These incorrect Doppler results are referred to as 'false positives'.
- ◆ If PAH is suspected from an echocardiogram, cardiac catheterization is usually performed because this is the only reliable test to make a definite diagnosis of PAH.

Echocardiography also tells us whether the right heart is larger than it should be and whether it is working normally. Therefore, we use several pieces of information from echocardiography to help us decide whether a patient is likely or unlikely to have PAH.

What does it involve?

The test is available in nearly all hospitals and is also done in primary care (GP surgeries and health centres). The scan is completely harmless and takes about 30 minutes.

The patient lies on their left side in a darkened room (so that the technician or doctor can see the monitor screen). You are connected with sticky electrode pads to an ECG. Ultrasound jelly is put on your chest, and the scan probe is pressed on the chest, over the ribs, and under the left breast. This can be a little tender. The heart is scanned and then the flow of blood through the heart and lungs is measured with a Doppler scan. You can see your heart on the screen. The sound of the blood circulating around the heart and lungs can be heard through the machine as a whooshing noise. Various measurements are taken and the results are sent to the PAH clinic or may be discussed with you at the time.

Lung function testing
What it tells us

If the history and initial investigations suggest a lung problem, lung function testing is a good way of finding out whether the lung disease is sufficiently severe to explain the breathlessness. The lung function tests measures a lot of other things as well, for example the speed at which you can breathe out.

People with *chronic bronchitis and asthma* cannot breathe out air quickly because their airways are narrowed and constricted. These conditions are grouped together and called *airways disease*. Another smoking-related disease is emphysema, which increases the size of the lungs by damaging the small air sacs and making it difficult for oxygen to get into the blood. This shows up on lung function tests as increased lung volumes. These conditions are common, and some PAH patients may have smoked in the past. It is important to find out whether PAH patients also have airways disease because we can treat this with puffers (inhalers), which improve their breathing.

In PAH, the main problem is inefficient uptake of oxygen because of reduced blood supply to the air sacs. In some types of PAH the reduction in gas exchange (also called the *transfer factor*, referring to gas transfer across the air sac wall) is much more than one would expect from consideration of all the other things we measure. We refer to this as 'disproportionate'. The gas transfer in a patient with PAH due to connective tissue disease is less than 50% of what we would expect in a normal person. However, in many patients with PAH the lung function tests are almost normal despite the patient being very breathless.

A minority of PAH patients whose PAH is linked to systemic sclerosis may also have *lung fibrosis (scarring)*. Lung function tests help us to decide whether patients have lung fibrosis and, if so, how severe it is. We also use lung scanning to help us decide how severe lung fibrosis is.

If the only major problem a breathless person has on lung function testing is a 'disproportionately' low transfer factor and all the other results from the lung function tests are normal or almost normal (no signs of asthma, bronchitis, or emphysema, or signs of that their lungs are 'small'), connective-tissue disease-associated PAH should be considered.

What is involved?

Compared with other tests you may have, lung function tests require you to do your bit! When you arrive, the tester will measure your weight and height. If they cannot measure your height (if you are in a wheelchair, for example), they will measure your arm span, which gives them a guide to your height.

This test requires you to blow through a mouthpiece or snorkel, possibly several times, for all you are worth into a special machine that measures the speed with which you can empty your lungs. If you wear dentures and they are loose, you might need to take them out when you blow into the machine. If you are breathing through your nose, and this is affecting your breathing test, you may be asked to wear a nose-clip. Needless to say, getting the maximum performance out of everyone requires a special sort of person—someone with sergeant-major qualities!

Spirometry is the first lung function test done. It measures how much and how quickly you can move air out of your lungs. For this test, you breathe into a mouthpiece attached to a recording device (spirometer).

You will also be asked to breathe in a special gas (a harmless amount of carbon monoxide). This allows the lung function machine to measure the total air capacity of your lungs (called the total lung capacity) and the efficiency with which gas can move into the blood. It may not be possible to measure certain things like the transfer factor if a patient is very breathless and cannot blow very hard.

Occasionally, the tester might ask you to sit in a booth which looks a bit like a small see-through shower cubicle. The door will be closed and the test will be done while you sit inside. This will help your tester obtain more detailed results.

The tests should take between 30 minutes and one hour. However, if you are very breathless, they may take longer. You won't be rushed through. Do your best.

Tests for home oxygen
What they tell us

If your breathing is very bad, you may have 'respiratory failure'. This means that your lungs are not delivering enough oxygen to the blood. It can also mean that they are also unable to expel waste gases such as carbon dioxide. If this is the case, you may need long-term home oxygen.

What is involved?

To test for respiratory failure a specialist will check your blood gases on two occasions about 2–3 weeks apart when you are reasonably well. If your oxygen is low, your blood gases will be checked again while you are breathing in extra oxygen through your nose. The oxygen is delivered by small see-through tubes known as nasal cannulae. The chest specialist can then work out how much oxygen you need to improve your levels.

At home the oxygen will be delivered from an oxygen concentrator—a machine (the size of a small refrigerator) which takes in air and produces oxygen. Generally people use concentrators for 15 or more hours per day, every day.

It is possible to buy portable oxygen concentrators or get small oxygen cylinders to take out of the house. Your doctor will order the oxygen for you from your local supplier and will check at least twice yearly that your concentrator is giving you enough oxygen and that the oxygen level in your blood is satisfactory.

Fitness to fly test
What it tells us

This test checks if it is safe for you to travel by plane. The tester measures how much oxygen is in your blood using an oximeter. If your blood oxygen level falls below 90% when the oxygen pressure falls, you should breathe in oxygen during the flight.

What is involved?

You wear a mask and breathe normally. The air you breathe through the mask will have a lower concentration of oxygen than normal air, as in a flight. The test lasts for 20 minutes.

If there is enough oxygen in your blood, you are fit to fly. If not, the specialist will repeat the test with a higher concentration of oxygen until the level of oxygen in your blood has reached an acceptable level.

The specialist will then give you a letter for the airline stating that you require oxygen on the flight and how much you need to have. You will need to check that the airline is able to provide oxygen and whether they will charge you for it before you book your flight. The fitness to fly test is valid for up to 3 months before you travel. The Pulmonary Hypertension Association (PHA) is very helpful and will give you all the practical advice you need.

The six-minute walk test
What it tells us

When we exercise, it has an effect on our breathing. The more exercise we do, the more oxygen our body needs. In PAH there is a problem with gas exchange, and so PAH patients cannot walk as much as normal people and this is typically the first thing that they notice. They become breathless much more quickly than normal, particularly when walking up inclines or stairs.

Many patients find it difficult to describe or measure how far and how fast they can walk. We need to know if patients are getting better and responding to treatment or not. We also need to know if patients not on treatment are deteriorating and should now be treated with PAH medication.

Patients who can walk more than 450 metres up and down the corridor in 6 minutes are doing well. We compare the distance patients walk and like to see the distance increase or at least remain stable.

> The distance PAH patients walk in 6 minutes is another piece of the jigsaw of information we use to decide on the treatments we offer.

What is involved?

The six-minute walk test is part of the consultation and is done either before or after you see the doctor and nurses. To check your breathing, the tester will ask you to do some exercise and take measurements while you are exercising, and afterwards.

We check the oxygen level in your blood using an oximeter on a finger or earlobe. You then walk at a comfortable pace up and down the corridor. We measure the distance walked in 6 minutes timed by a stopwatch. We re-measure the oxygen content in your blood. We then ask you to fill in a form describing how you felt and how breathless you were the end of the test. This is called the Borg scale.

People who cannot walk cannot do the test. People who have problems with their feet and legs may also not be able to do the test at all, or may be restricted because of these other problems rather than breathlessness. You should tell the PAH specialist why you think you have to stop walking. Is it breathlessness or another problem?

Most PAH centres use the six-minute walk distance, but there are other ways that we measure how much a patient can do.

- ◆ Walking at your own pace for 6 minutes, taking as many rests as you need.
- ◆ Walking on a treadmill, while the tester monitors your heart and lungs.
- ◆ Doing a test on an exercise bike. This is done occasionally if the doctors need more detailed information about your breathing. Usually you will be asked to breathe through a mouthpiece while you cycle. The amount of oxygen you breathe in and the carbon dioxide you breathe out are measured, as well as your breathing rate, your pulse, and sometimes your blood gases.

Ventilation–perfusion lung scan (V–Q scan) to detect blood clots in the lungs (pulmonary emboli)
What it tells us

Blood clots form in the legs, or in the big veins in the pelvis, following long periods of immobility (e.g. during frequent long-haul flights or after major operations). Patients are now routinely treated with blood-thinning injections after high-risk operations to prevent clots. Clots are more likely to occur in people who are very overweight, dehydrated (alcohol and hot climates can cause this), or inactive which slows down the circulation of blood in the legs.

A blood clot (thrombosis) in the leg (deep vein thrombosis (DVT)) results in swelling and pain in the calf. The clot can be seen using ultrasound. The danger of a DVT is that it can break off from the wall of the vein, and travel up through the right side of the heart to the lung arteries. This is called a *pulmonary embolus*. If the clot is very large, it can obstruct blood flow to the lungs, causing collapse, chest pain, and shortness of breath. This can be very dangerous. This is a medical emergency and patients should go directly to hospital. Smaller clots may cause only mild symptoms or no symptoms.

Some patients notice breathlessness quite some time after the pulmonary embolus. The reason for this is not clear, but it is due to PAH. This is called chronic thromboembolic disease associated pulmonary hypertension (CTED-PH). These patients need lifelong treatment with warfarin. They may also benefit from a major operation to remove the clots from the lungs. This is called thromboendarterectomy (cutting or extracting the clot from the inside of the vessel).

What is involved

A *ventilation–perfusion scan* is actually two tests, done either separately or at the same time.

Normally, the blood supply (perfusion) to each part of the lung should 'match' the amount of air we breathe in (ventilation).

If the blood supply to a part or parts of the lungs does not match the amount of ventilation we call this a 'ventilation–perfusion mismatch'. The most important cause of a mismatch is clots in the lung arteries. Blood clots do *not* affect the volume of air reaching the lungs, only the blood supply.

If a patient has severe lung disease, it may be difficult to interpret the scan because both ventilation and perfusion may be affected by the lung condition.

You are given both *inhaled* and *injected* radioactive material (radio-isotopes) to measure air entry into the blood *(ventilation)* and blood supply *(perfusion)* to all areas of the lungs.

During the perfusion scan, radioactive albumin is injected into a vein, usually in the arm or at the back of the hand. You are placed on a movable table that is under the arm of a scanner. The machine scans your lungs as blood flows through them to find the location of the radioactive particles.

During the ventilation scan, you breathe in radioactive gas through a mask while you are sitting or lying on a table under the scanner arm.

You do not need to stop eating (fast), eat a special diet, or take any medications before the test.

A chest X-ray is usually done before or after a ventilation–perfusion scan.

You will sign a consent form and wear a hospital gown or comfortable clothing that does not have metal fasteners.

The table may feel hard or cold. You may feel a sharp prick while the material is injected into the vein for the perfusion part of the scan.

The mask used during the ventilation scan may make you feel nervous about being in a small space (claustrophobia). You must lie still during the scan.

The radio-isotope injection does not usually cause discomfort.

Normal results

All parts of both lungs should take up the radio-isotope evenly. The amount of isotope inhaled should be matched by a similar amount of injected isotope reaching the lung via the pulmonary arteries and their branches.

What abnormal results mean

If the lungs take up below-normal amounts of radio-isotope during a ventilation or perfusion scan, it may be due to:

◆ airway obstruction

◆ a problem with blood flow (such as clots in the lung arteries)

◆ lung damage from smoking

◆ pneumonia

◆ reduced breathing and ventilation ability.

Risks of a ventilation–perfusion scan

Radiation risks are about the same as for X-rays. No radiation is released from the scanner. Instead, it detects radiation and converts it into an image. There is a small exposure to radiation from the radio-isotope. The radio-isotopes used during scans are short-lived. All of the radiation leaves the body in a few days. However, as with any radiation exposure, caution is advised for pregnant or breast-feeding women. In rare cases, a person may develop an allergy to the radio-isotope.

Considerations

A pulmonary ventilation–perfusion scan may be a lower-risk alternative to pulmonary angiography for evaluating disorders of the lung blood supply. This test may not provide an absolute diagnosis, especially in people with lung disease. Other tests may be needed to confirm or rule out the findings of a pulmonary ventilation–perfusion scan.

Cardiac catheterization

What it tells us

The information is used to diagnose and treat conditions which, if ignored, can lead to death and debility. Therefore it is a very important test. A cardiac catheter test is sometimes called an angiogram but, strictly speaking, an angiogram (*angio*, blood vessel; *gram*, picture) is an X-ray picture of blood vessels anywhere in the body. Angiograms are often done at the same time as the catheter test.

The only way to be sure that a patient has, or has not got PAH, and to see if they are responding to treatment, is to measure the pressures in the lung arteries and the heart with a tube. The tube is called a catheter.

For diagnosis, a catheter test is done only in patients who are likely to have PAH or in whom it is important to exclude it if the other tests are borderline.

For monitoring purposes, it is also done to see if there have been any changes in the pressures in the lungs, in the heart, and in the resistance to blood flow through the lungs in patients who have started new treatments or who feel they are deteriorating.

A patient has PAH if the mean pressure in the lung arteries is 25 mmHg or more, where the high pressure is not caused by back pressure from the left heart or very high flow rates through the lung arteries.

We measure pressures in the lung arteries (pulmonary artery pressure), the lung capillaries (pulmonary wedge pressure), and the right heart (right atrial and right ventricular pressure). We also measure the amount of blood that the heart is pumping around the body per minute. This is the *cardiac output*. With these figures, we can work out the *resistance to blood flow in the lungs* (pulmonary vascular resistance).

The test can and is repeated to see how patients respond to treatment. It is may also be done to exclude PAH in a patient who has a borderline echocardiogram result.

We can also take blood samples through the catheter to measure the oxygen content of the blood in various positions in the *right heart*. Using a different catheter inserted in an artery, we can take blood samples to measure the oxygen content from the chambers of the *left heart*. This information tells us if there are any *holes in the heart* or other types of shunt, and we can work out how serious the shunt is. A shunt is suspected from the clinical examination and the echocardiography and Doppler test.

Neither normal nor abnormal lung pressures

Some patients have a mean pulmonary artery pressure of less than 25 mmHg but are not completely 'normal'. Their mean pulmonary artery pressure may be between 20 and 24 mmHg. This is higher than the normal level of 18 mmHg, but not quite high enough for a diagnosis of PAH. These patients, who are not completely normal and do not have PAH, may be at a very early stage of PAH. They need to be monitored very carefully, at least once a year, to see if they develop PAH so that they can be treated promptly if and when necessary.

What is involved?

The tests are done as day cases. The test should be painless, but you might feel a jab and stinging sensation when the local anaesthetic is injected into the skin. The test takes less than 30 minutes.

Tests are done in a cardiac catheter laboratory—an X-ray room. There is a very skilled team of nurses, a radiographer, and a cardiac physiologist working with the doctor doing the test. Some doctors are cardiologists and others are lung specialists. The test is usually explained by both the doctor and the nurses when you come to clinic, and again before you sign a consent form when you come in to hospital.

You should not eat or drink for 3 hours before the test. If you are taking *metformin*, this should be stopped 3 days before the test. *Warfarin* should be stopped 3 days before the test. You do not need to stop *aspirin*. If you have had pulmonary emboli, you should take injections of an anticoagulant called *clexane* (or something similar) for the days when you are not taking warfarin so that your blood remains thin.

Risks

There is a 1 in 1000 risk of death, arrhythmia, or lung or leg damage. This is why we do the test only when it is really necessary to find out if a patient has or does not have PAH, in patients who deteriorate to see if the reason is because their lung pressure has increased, and to see if patients are responding to treatment.

Groin or neck vein?

The test can be done from either the groin vein or the neck vein. There are pros and cons with each approach. The advantages of doing the test from the groin is that in addition to measuring the heart pressures, another tube can be inserted into the artery next to the vein to see if there are any blockages or narrowing in the heart (coronary arteries). This test is called a *coronary angiogram*.

The advantage of using the neck vein is that the catheter most commonly used was designed to be used from the neck (although experienced and skilled operators can use it very easily from the groin) and it is easier to manipulate from the neck than the groin. However, if the right heart catheter test is being done from the neck and a coronary angiogram also needs to be done, this would be less convenient. A coronary angiogram can be done from the groin or the wrist. The patient may need to be invited back for this additional procedure.

Vasodilator testing

A vasodilator (*vaso*, vessel; *dilator*, open or widen) test is done as part of the right heart catheter test. It tells us if a patient who has PAH might respond to medications which lower the pressure by relaxing and widening the tight constricted lung arteries.

A drug is used to relax the lung arteries, either nitric oxide (which you breathe in) or prostacyclin which is injected into a vein very slowly and carefully to see if the lung pressure falls by a certain amount. If the pressure does fall (and this occurs in only a minority of patients with PAH), this tells us that a large part of the high pressure is due to spasm of the lung arteries, rather than thickening or overgrowth of cells in the lung artery wall. This is called a 'positive' vasodilator response. Some patients may feel light-headed or develop a headache during the test because of the medication used. If there is no fall in the lung pressure, this is called a 'negative vasodilator test'.

Those who respond are treated with tablets called *calcium antagonists (diltiazem or amlodipine)*, which relax the muscle of the lung arteries, increasing the blood supply to the lungs.

Coronary angiogram
What it tells us

Some PAH patients have coronary heart disease (furring up or blockages in the heart arteries). It is important to know if some of their symptoms are caused by a lack of blood and oxygen supply to their left heart muscle. Coronary angiography is the most accurate way to see if a patient has narrowing or blockages in their heart arteries. If they do and they have bad symptoms of angina which are not controlled with tablets and control of their risk factors (weight loss, diet, stopping smoking, control of blood pressure and diabetes, exercise, and treating stress), the symptoms can be treated by improving the blood supply to the left heart muscle. This can be done by either opening and widening the heart artery (*angioplasty*), usually by implanting a stent, or bypassing the narrowing or blockage with an operation (*bypass surgery*). Some patients are treated with both angioplasty and heart bypass.

 Coronary heart disease is *not* more common in PAH than in people who do not have PAH, unless the patient with PAH has risk factors for coronary heart disease (systemic high blood pressure, smoking, family history, high cholesterol, diabetes).

What is involved?

Coronary angiography can conveniently be done at the same time as the right heart catheter test. Coronary angioplasty can also often done at the same time as the coronary angiogram. Coronary angiography is done most commonly from the groin artery, using local anaesthetic, which might sting. The risks and the preparation beforehand are similar to a right heart catheter test.

The contrast injected into the heart arteries gets into the circulation. This can cause kidney damage, and so a kidney function blood test must be done before the coronary angiogram. Patients should not take *metformin* for 3 days before the test because these can also damage the kidneys. The contrast fluid contains iodine. Patients who know or think they have an iodine allergy should tell the person doing their angiogram, and they may be given antihistamines and hydrocortisone cortisone before the procedure.

The contrast fluid can make a minority of patients feel rather sick and flushed, and some patients also feel a funny feeling that they have 'wet themselves' if a large volume of contrast fluid is injected into the left heart pumping chamber.

This part may not be necessary because most patients would have had an echocardiogram before the catheter test.

The additional risk is bruising over the groin and, very occasionally, a lump or haematoma over the artery. Very rarely, the artery can develop a blow-out, or *aneurysm*, which is usually easily dealt with. These risks do not generally occur with a right heart catheter because the pressure in the veins is much lower than in the arteries.

Invasive pulmonary angiogram
What it tells us

Some PAH centres do this test, but others rely on non-invasive imaging of the lung circulation. Some centres do both. Invasive pulmonary angiography shows in great detail, the lung arteries and if there are blockages or other signs of blood clots in the lung arteries due to pulmonary emboli. This information is very helpful in deciding whether a patient would benefit from clot removal (thrombo-endarterectomy).

What is involved?

The test is usually done as part of the catheter test. A special catheter is inserted into either the neck vein or the groin vein. Under X-ray control, the tube is inserted into the right and left heart lung arteries, and contrast fluid is injected into the arteries of both lungs while pictures are taken. The risks of this test are similar to those of the catheter test.

High-resolution computed tomography (HRCT) lung scan
What it tells us

Nearly all hospitals in the UK now have CT scanners. CT scanning is a form of X-ray examination, but the radiation dose is higher than a chest X-ray.

CT scanning combines special X-ray equipment with sophisticated computers to produce multiple images or pictures of the inside of the body. These cross-sectional images of the area being studied can then be examined on a computer monitor or printed.

CT scans of internal organs, bone, soft tissue, and blood vessels provide greater clarity and reveal more details than regular X-ray examinations. CT of the chest is used:

- to provide more detailed information about abnormalities seen on a chest X-ray
- to help diagnose the cause of clinical signs or symptoms of disease of the chest, such as cough, shortness of breath, chest pain, or fever

◆ to detect and evaluate the extent of tumours that arise in the chest, or tumours that have spread there from other parts of the body.

chest CT can demonstrate various lung disorders, such as:

◆ lung cancer

◆ pneumonia and other chest infections

◆ emphysema

◆ bronchiectasis

◆ inflammation or other diseases of the lining covering the lung *(pleura)*

◆ diffuse interstitial lung disease.

The last of these is important in PAH because lung scarring (fibrosis or interstitial lung disease) can cause and contribute to PAH. HRCT tells us how severe the fibrosis is and how much there is.

What is involved?

The CT scanner is a large box-like machine with a hole or short tunnel in the centre. You will lie on a narrow examination table that slides into and out of this tunnel. The X-ray tube rotates around you. The computer workstation that processes the imaging information is located in a separate room, where the radiographer operates the scanner and monitors your examination.

You should wear comfortable loose-fitting clothing, and you may be asked to wear a gown. Metal objects including jewelry, metal-framed glasses, dentures, and hairpins may affect the CT images, and should be left at home or removed prior to your scan. You may also be asked to remove hearing aids and removable dental work.

The PAH specialist would have informed the radiographer about your medical history, but you may be asked about any recent illnesses or other medical conditions, and if you have a history of heart disease, asthma, diabetes, kidney disease, or thyroid problems. Women should always inform their physician and the radiographer if there is any possibility that they are pregnant

The radiation dose is higher than a chest X-ray and so these scans should be done only if it is important to investigate serious lung problems.

Contrast-enhanced computed tomographic pulmonary angiography (CTPA) for blood clots
What it tells us

A CTPA scan shows the blood vessels (arteries and veins) in the chest. The severity of breathlessness depends on the number of blocked arteries and where the blockages are. A CTPA scan tells us if there are clots (pulmonary emboli) in the lungs, where they are, how many lung arteries have been blocked, and whether an operation to remove the blood clots (thombo-endarterectomy) is likely to help. Some PAH units also do invasive pulmonary angiography.

What is involved?

CT examinations are generally painless, fast, and easy. An iodine-based contrast fluid is injected into a vein shortly before scanning begins.

The only discomfort is the needle inserted into a vein in your arm or the back of your hand. If you find it difficult lying still, are claustrophobic, or have pain when lying still, you should tell the radiographer, who may offer you a small dose of sedative. You may have a warm flushed sensation during the injection of the contrast fluid, and a metallic taste in your mouth that lasts for a few minutes.

You will be alone in the examination room during the CT scan. The radiographer can hear and see you from the side room during the scan. You lie still on your back on the X-ray table, which moves through the scanner quite quickly while numerous X-ray pictures are taken of your lungs. A computer processes these pictures and creates a picture of your lungs and the lung arteries. CT imaging is sometimes compared to looking into a loaf of bread by cutting it into thin slices.

You may be asked to hold your breath during the scanning. This is to avoid blurring of the images while breathing. The actual CT scanning takes less than 30 seconds and the entire process is usually completed within 30 minutes. You may be asked to wait for a few minutes to make sure the pictures are satisfactory. After the scan drink plenty of fluid to flush the contrast fluid out of your body.

A radiologist will send a report to the doctor who requested the scan.

Risks of CT scanning

Unlike MRI, CT can be performed if you have an implanted medical device (pacemaker, metal prosthesis) of any kind.

No radiation remains in a patient's body after a CT examination. X-rays used in CT scans usually have no side-effects. The risk of cancer is negligible. The benefit of an accurate diagnosis far outweighs the risk. The effective radiation dose from this procedure is about the same as the average person receives from background radiation in 2 years. Women should always inform their physician and the radiographer if there is any possibility that they are pregnant. In general, CT scanning is not recommended for pregnant women unless medically necessary because of potential risk to the baby.

You may be asked not to eat or drink anything for a few hours beforehand, as contrast material will be used. You should inform the radiographer of any medications you are taking and if you have any allergies. If you have a known allergy to contrast material, or 'dye', your doctor may prescribe medications to reduce the risk of an allergic reaction.

In order to see clots in the lung arteries, an iodine-containing fluid (contrast fluid) is injected rapidly into a vein, in the arm or back of the hand, while the scanner takes pictures.

The risk of serious allergic reaction to contrast materials that contain iodine is extremely rare, and radiology departments are well equipped to deal with them. All tests that involve contrast can aggravate damaged kidneys. If your kidney function is poor you will be given fluids (usually bicarbonate) around the time of your X-ray.

Magnetic resonance imaging (MRI) with or without contrast

What it tells us

An MRI scan with the injection of contrast fluid tells us whether arteries almost anywhere in the body, including the heart and lung arteries, are narrowed or blocked and how severe the narrowing is. It is also used to detect tears in the main artery in the tummy (aorta).

MRI of the heart also tells us about the structure of the heart and if it is working normally. In PAH it is sometimes used in addition to echocardiography to monitor the heart's response to treatment of PAH.

What is involved?

The scan is similar to a CT scan. The scan cannot be done if you have a pace-maker, but can be done if you have a metal stent in a heart artery.

Abdominal ultrasound

What it tells us

This ultrasound scan of the tummy tells us about the size of the liver, kidneys, and spleen, and if there are tumours in the abdomen. It shows cirrhosis or other damage to the liver which is a rare cause of PAH.

What is involved?

You lie on your back, ultrasound jelly is put on your tummy, and a probe is pressed on the skin and moved around to look at various organs in the abdomen. It is quick and completely harmless. It does not involve X-rays. You may be asked not to eat or drink for a few hours before the scan.

10

Clinical trials and evidence-based medicine

➡️ Key points

- It takes several years for a new drug to be licensed. Each drug is tested carefully in clinical trials to provide evidence that the drug is safe and that it works. This is called evidence-based medicine.

- Further advances can be made only with the help and participation of patients in clinical trials. These are organized and run by your PAH centre.

Discovering new treatments

Once the mechanism or cause of a medical illness is known, scientists and doctors can design a drug to cure it. Antibiotics are developed in this way. Thyroxine, insulin, and other hormone replacement drugs are other examples of this logical scientific approach to treatment—find the cause of a condition and treat it.

Some drugs are discovered to work by chance. A drug may have been tried in one condition, but caused an unexpected but useful side-effect which was beneficial for another problem (e.g. phosphodiesterase-5 inhibitors). Some are manufactured to block the actions of naturally occurring but harmful chemicals (e.g. endothelin receptor antagonists (ERAs)). Others are manufactured to increase the amount of naturally occurring and helpful chemicals (e.g. prostanoids).

Discovering new drugs to treat PAH

Sildenafil (Viagra) was initially used in trials for systemic hypertension and angina. It was ineffective in these condition, but men found that they developed erections. Viagra is now used to treat erectile dysfunction. Viagra works by prolonging and increasing the action of an important chemical called nitric oxide which opens up arteries and keeps them open (vasodilator). Nitric oxide is produced by the lining cells (endothelium) of arteries. The beneficial effects of nitric oxide are short-lived because it is destroyed by an enzyme called phosphodiesterase-5 (PDE-5). Sildenafil inhibits the action of PDE-5 and so prolongs the beneficial effects of nitric oxide.

The lung arteries in PAH are narrowed and go into spasm or constrict. It seemed logical to use Viagra in PAH to see if it helped to keep the lung arteries open. Trials were performed and Viagra was found to work. It is now one of the three main groups of drugs that we use to treat PAH. There are other similar drugs which work in the same way, prolonging the action of nitric oxide; interestingly, when used in PAH, they do not appear to affect penile erection.

Endothelin is a naturally occurring chemical which causes thickening and constriction of the walls of lung arteries. Patients with PAH have excess endothelin. Drugs blocking the action of endothelin (endothelin receptor antagonists) are used in PAH. This is an example of a drug used to block the actions of a substance which contributes to narrowed lung arteries.

Prostacyclin is another naturally occurring chemical which widens arteries. Drugs like prostacyclin have been manufactured (prostanoids) and are used to treat PAH. This is an example of manufacturing drugs similar to a beneficial naturally produced substance.

Clinical trials produce evidence-based medicine

Patients and doctors want treatments that are safe and effective. This information can be provided only by painstaking tests and trials of drugs. This research takes several years and costs a considerable amount of money.

Modern medicine is all about prescribing tablets and other treatments which have been proved in clinical trials (trials done in patients) to be better than a *placebo* (Latin 'to please'), i.e. an inactive substance not thought to have any effect on the condition.

In order to find out if a drug works and is better than placebo, a *placebo-controlled* or *controlled* trial is necessary. The drug has to be compared with placebo in a large number of patients with a specified condition, *randomly* allocated to the active drug or placebo. To ensure that neither the patients nor the doctors are biased against the placebo or in favour of the drug when they assess the patients' responses to drug and placebo, the placebo is manufactured to look exactly like the active drug. Neither the doctors nor the patients know or can see which tablet is the placebo and which tablet is the active drug. Both parties are 'blinded'. This trial design is called a *double-blind randomized placebo-controlled trial*. The results from this trial design provide the most powerful and reliable evidence about whether a drug is safe, if it really works, and how well it works.

If it does work well and is better than placebo, then we have the evidence we need to prescribe the drug. This is 'evidence-based medicine'.

Can we prescribe new drugs simply on the evidence?

Evidence-based medicine is important because it helps to justify using expensive medications. However, this evidence alone may not always be enough for the healthcare managers responsible for paying for the medications to approve our requests to them to pay for your drugs.

They may want to know, amongst other considerations, how many patients would need to be treated and for how long, and at what cost, for the drug to result in a meaningful cost-effective improvement in survival, reduced disability, and reduction in time spent in hospital. Like clinicians, they want to be convinced that the new drug is better, more effective, and safer than another less expensive drug. Does the evidence from the trials justify its use? Is it worth the cost and the price of any side-effects?

Consensus treatment decisions

PAH clinicians are advocates for patients. They try to give them the best possible care. They work closely with commissioning agencies (currently called primary care trusts (PCTs)) to try to secure the best treatments for patients. PAH clinicians have a responsibility to give the best possible care to their patients, but they also have to be mindful of the available resources for healthcare. In new fields of medicine, where there is comparatively less evidence on which to base treatment decisions, clinicians also have a responsibility to use their clinical experience, which is influenced by various factors, and also to make decisions after detailed discussions with other experts. This is called consensus management, and is important in current PAH management. Patients have to be treated with what we believe to be the most appropriate treatments while we await the results of clinical trials.

Combination therapy: costs and is it better than one treatment?

It seems reasonable that patients who deteriorate on one form of treatment may benefit from adding in another drug which works in a different but complementary way. Combining drugs in this way is called *combination therapy*. This is quite a new approach because the opportunity to use combination therapy had to await the arrival of new treatments. However, PCTs and similar agencies elsewhere may not be convinced that it is cost effective. There are also issues about safety and drug interactions, and so it is not yet clear whether there are definite advantages.

Before starting combination therapy, the PAH team will need to know if the patient is deteriorating or not responding satisfactorily to treatment and has, or is at risk of, right heart failure. Each case is carefully considered and the options discussed with the patient and their family.

If it is decided that the patient might benefit, and the patient agrees, they may be invited to participate in a clinical trial testing whether the additional drug is beneficial and safe. Alternatively, an application has to be made to their PCT.

Combination therapy is expensive. In the UK, endothelin receptor antagonists cost around £20 000 per year, sildenafil costs £10 000 per year, and prostanoids cost up to £60 000 per year.

This underlines the importance of a constructive and mutually sympathetic relationship and understanding between commissioners and government drug funding agencies, and PAH specialists. Senior managers in government funding agencies need to be constantly updated on the results of clinical trials so that they are able to be flexible in their drug approval policies.

There is some evidence from trials that combination therapy provides a small but definite advantage compared with using only one treatment. Trials have shown a small improvement (20 metres) in the distance patients can walk in 6 minutes compared with placebo, and in most trials they also prevent the PAH worsening over time. Despite the currently thin evidence in favour of combination therapy, PAH specialists feel compelled to do everything they can to help patients. The results of further studies will help us decide on the value of combination therapy, but PAH specialists intuitively believe that it should benefit patients.

Trials in PAH: what are the important questions about new drugs?

In PAH trials comparing a new drug with placebo, the information we want to know about the new drug includes the following.

◆ Do patients live longer?

◆ Are they able to do more and walk further and more quickly?

◆ Do patients feel better?

◆ Does it improve and lower the pressure in the lung arteries and the heart?

◆ Does it improve the heart function and lower the resistance to blood flow in the lungs?

◆ Does it slow down progression of the disease?

◆ What are its side-effects and its effects on the blood? How safe is it?

Trials of new PAH drugs are important

PAH is an uncommon disease. Compared with other much more common conditions, such as systemic hypertension, there are not many patients who can participate in trials. Therefore PAH units around the world (multicentre) collaborate in clinical trials so that there are enough patients in the trial to draw firm conclusions. The more patients in the trial, the better; this makes either a positive or negative result more likely to be reliable.

The aim is to test new drugs to see whether they are safe, whether they work, and whether they are better than older drugs. Ideally, the trials should test a new drug in a specific type of PAH because it is by no means certain that all types of PAH respond in the same way to the same drug.

Most PAH patients are on treatment. Because of the risks of them deteriorating if they stopped the treatment or switched to placebo, it is considered unethical to ask them to stop all their treatment to participate in a placebo-controlled trial. One way around this is to add either the new drug or placebo on top of the PAH treatment they are taking.

Placebos and complementary therapies

A placebo is a harmless tablet or other form of treatment which does not contain an active ingredient or action to improve a condition. However, we have known for many years that placebos 'work' and can make people feel better.

The power of a reassuring and comforting consultation or, for some, a religious experience, and, for many, a holiday, is well known. Many people with all sorts of conditions (e.g. headaches, aches and pains, tummy upsets, stress and anxiety) feel better with what traditionally trained doctors consider to be untested placebos. Interestingly, even people with quite serious conditions, such as heart failure, feel better and walk further if treated with placebo but, unlike effective drugs, these do not improve the underlying condition or make people live longer. Massage, aromatherapy, and various other 'complementary' forms of treatment certainly make some people feel better.

The mechanisms of various psychological therapies are difficult to understand, but many people find them very helpful. Herbal remedies cannot be subjected to the same rigorous trials as traditional medicines. They are not quite the same as other forms of complementary medicine because they contain various substances which do exert effects on the body. Interestingly, one of the best heart tablets, digoxin, which we have used for centuries to treat heart failure and which we use in most people with PAH, is derived from the foxglove plant, and there are other examples of herbal and plant remedies. The danger with herbal remedies lies in the fact that the amount of active ingredients changes from batch to batch, so even if active ingredients are present, one cannot know that the right amount is being taken.

Complementary medications and other drug interactions with PAH medications

Some PAH patients like complementary therapies, and with some therapies, such as homeopathy, there is no risk as long as effective treatments are also taken and worsening symptoms are not ignored while alternative approaches are explored.

Various other drugs can interfere with PAH medications. PAH medications interact with each other and with other treatments. These are called drug interactions and can be dangerous. That is why it is really important for you to tell your PAH team about *every* tablet or medication you take in case it interacts with your PAH treatments. There is also a difference between what a patient is prescribed and what they actually take! Please tell your PAH specialist about *all* the medications and other treatments that you take.

Controlled trials in PAH

Compared with the treatment of other medical conditions (e.g. angina, systemic hypertension), PAH is a newcomer. This is because it is only recently that we have understood some of the mechanisms of why it occurs and only very recently that there have been drugs to treat it.

Other types of research in PAH
Comparing the outlook for PAH patients today with the past

We want to know if we are improving the care of patients with PAH. We need to know whether patients are doing better with modern treatments compared with older forms of treatment. It cannot be assumed that just because a treatment is 'new' it is necessarily better. We monitor outcomes in groups of patients over long periods of time and enter the results of clinical assessments and tests in a national registry. This provides very useful information about how patients get on in real life and is different from a controlled drug trial.

The larger the group of patients and longer the observation period, the more helpful is the study. Therefore we assess how a group of patients with a particular type of PAH, treated with certain medications, fares compared with a group of similar patients who were treated in the past with older forms of treatment. This is done by carefully monitoring patients over a long period of time and seeing what happens to them. This is sometimes called 'outcomes research' or an observational study.

We record and collect a lot of information on all our patients every time we see them in clinic or if they come for tests, including cardiac catheter tests done to record the pressures in the heart and lungs, or are admitted to hospital. These tests are done as part of routine clinical practice and do not require sanction from an ethics committee. We are not doing anything over and above what is required as part of the patients' treatment.

Not all of the following tests are done every time we see patients. We only do the tests we feel are necessary for a particular patient at the time. We record the results of the following:

◆ clinical examination, including their exercise tolerance (what sort of activities they are able to do before getting breathless)

◆ six-minute walk test (how far they can walk on the flat in 6 minutes)

- blood tests
- breathing tests
- heart ultrasound (echocardiogram)
- chest X-rays
- electrical recording of the heart (ECG)
- scans of the heart and lungs
- cardiac catheter tests.

11

Supportive treatments for PAH

→ Key points

- Supportive treatments include the blood thinner (anticoagulant) warfarin, water tablets (diuretics) to get rid of excess water caused by some of the PAH medications (endothelin receptor antagonists) and heart failure, oxygen, and digoxin to control the heart rhythm.

- They are called supportive or background therapies or treatments because they do not directly affect the lung arteries, only the consequences of PAH and its effects on the right heart.

- Although supportive treatments have not been subjected to controlled clinical trials like other PAH treatments, from clinical experience it makes sense to use them.

- Patients should *not* take warfarin if the risks of bleeding outweigh its benefits.

- Only patients with a low oxygen level need oxygen.

- Regular checks of your blood count, kidney function, and clotting state (international normalized ratio (INR)) are important.

Supportive treatments help control symptoms of PAH

Supportive treatments are used to control some of the problems caused by PAH and heart failure. Unlike the targeted therapies, which have been shown in controlled trials to benefit PAH patients, there is no trial evidence that supportive therapies improve survival, but PAH specialists believe that they should be used.

- **Diuretics** are necessary to treat water retention caused by heart failure and some of the targeted therapies.

- **Oxygen** increases the oxygen level in patients with a low oxygen level.

- **Digoxin** is used in left heart failure because it strengthens the heart and also slows down the heart rate and makes it more efficient. It is reasonable to use it in right heart failure for the same reasons.

◆ PAH patients are at risk of blood clots in the lung arteries because of the slow flow of blood through the arteries and the increased clotting tendency in PAH. **Warfarin** (a blood thinner) reduces the risk of clots forming in the lung arteries.

So, although there may not be evidence from clinical controlled trials that these supportive treatments work, their use makes sense. They are safe, are effective in controlling symptoms, and are not expensive. Although these treatments do not affect the thickening of the lung artery wall in PAH, they do prevent and treat the consequences of the condition and its effects on the right heart.

Diuretics

How do they work?

Diuretics or water tablets have been used for all types of heart failure since they were first discovered in the early twentieth century. There are now several very good and effective 'loop diuretics' which are used to treat and prevent water retention caused by right heart failure and some PAH treatments. They work by making the kidneys get rid of salt and water from the body.

Diuretics are the most important drugs used to treat fluid accumulation in the feet, legs, and tummy of patients with *right heart failure*. They are also the key drugs used to get rid of excess fluid in the lungs caused by *left heart failure*, which is most commonly caused by systemic high blood pressure and furring up of the heart arteries (angina and heart attacks) and also occurs in more elderly patients with a stiff heart muscle.

The choice of diuretic will be made by your PAH specialist, but furosemide or bumetanide, possibly combined with a different type of diuretic called spironolactone, are the ones most commonly used. Occasionally, a small dose of metolazone may be used for a short time in patients who do not respond to the other diuretics.

What you should do

You might wonder, given how inconvenient these tablets are for patients (always running to the loo), why no study has been performed to find out what effect they have on survival. Why are diuretics used if there is no solid evidence? First, swollen ankles are uncomfortable, and when severe can lead to sores on the skin of the leg which can become infected. Secondly, the heart is known to be more efficient when it is not too fluid-logged. Thirdly, accumulation of fluid in the abdomen (tummy) can make it difficult to eat enough and to avoid losing weight. Therefore diuretics are used because they make people feel more comfortable and can easily be shown to stop some nasty complications of heart failure. Millions of people around the world take diuretics quite safely, but only if they are necessary.

Diuretics do not interfere with any of the usual medications prescribed for PAH.

You can take diuretics before or after meals. Take them in the morning and/or at lunchtime. If you take them at night, you will be up all night in the loo. If you are going out in the morning or will be travelling, take them when you get home. It may be OK for you to miss one dose, but you may feel breathless and get swollen feet and legs if you miss more than one or two doses.

Side-effects are very uncommon with moderate doses of diuretics.

It is very important to have your kidney function and electrolytes checked before you start and then at intervals while you take diuretics, because they may upset your kidney function and lower your electrolytes (sodium and potassium minerals).

You should not restrict the amount of water or other fluids you drink. Drink as much as you like, when you like. This is important if you are going to a hot climate.

Anticoagulants
How do they work?
Warfarin is a synthetic derivative of coumarin, a chemical found naturally in many plants, notably woodruff, and at lower levels in licorice, lavender, and various other species. Anticoagulants block the action of the clotting factor vitamin K in the liver, so that blood does not clot so quickly.

Anticoagulants were initially used in PAH because it was thought that the clots seen in the narrowed and thickened lung arteries were due to slow blood flow. Blood is more likely to clot when the flow in a blood vessel is slow. In PAH there is a tendency to increased clotting due to heart failure and immobility. There is also a defect in the body's ability to dissolve clots, and this increases a patient's tendency to clot. Finally, the clotting system has been shown to be activated in people with PAH, and blocking this has been shown experimentally to reduce the rate of lung vessel thickening.

There is evidence from two large registries that patients taking anticoagulants are more likely to survive longer than patients who don't take anticoagulants. The findings were from patients with idiopathic PAH. If it happens in idiopathic PAH, we believe that the same happens in the other forms of PAH.

Warfarin helps also helps to prevent clots blocking Hickman lines in patients treated with intravenous prostanoids (iloprost and trepositinil).

 All patients with PAH are advised to take life-long warfarin to reduce the risk of blood clots in the lungs, unless the risks of bleeding from warfarin outweigh its benefits.

Who should not take warfarin?

Patients with PAH associated with porto-pulmonary hypertension (PAH due to liver problems) should *not* take warfarin because their clotting system is likely to be disturbed by their liver disease. Their blood is already thin and they are more prone to bleeding from vessels in the gullet. Warfarin in patients with severe long-standing liver disease could cause life-threatening bleeding.

Some PAH patients have an irregular heart beat due to atrial fibrillation and may already be on warfarin for this reason.

What you should do

You will need regular blood tests, every 6 weeks or so, to check that the dose you are taking is safely thinning your blood. This test measures the *international normalized ratio (INR)* which should be between 2 and 3. The test is done either at your local hospital or at your GP health clinic. The best time to take warfarin is in the evening so that the level in your blood is stable by the time you have your blood test in the morning.

Many commonly used medications, and some foods, interact with warfarin. It is advisable not to have large alcohol binges. It is quite safe to have a glass of wine or a small glass of beer a day. Regular small doses of alcohol are not dangerous, and generally make people relaxed and stimulate the appetite. This is important in people who are unwell and lose weight. The warfarin dose can be adjusted to keep your INR within the right range. If your INR is too low, the warfarin dose will be increased and vice versa.

Endothelin receptor antagonists (ERAs) interact with warfarin. The dose of warfarin may need reducing after starting an ERA.

If you miss a dose, take the missed warfarin tablet with your usual tablet the following day.

Bring your yellow warfarin booklet with you to clinic. The PAH team often need to check that your INR is well controlled.

The INR in some patients is not easy to control. Some patients need very large doses to bring the INR up to the right range. This is nothing to worry about.

 Warfarin rarely cause side-effects apart from bleeding if too much is taken. If you feel more breathless, get chest pain, headache, palpitation, or any other side-effect, it is almost certainly *not* due to warfarin. If you think you have a side-effect, speak to your PAH team.

Consult your doctor immediately if you experience any of the following while on this medication:

* prolonged bleeding from cuts
* bleeding that does not stop by itself
* nose bleeds
* bleeding gums
* red or dark brown coloured urine
* for women, increased bleeding during periods (or any other vaginal bleeding).

Warfarin is damaging to the fetus, but people with PAH should avoid pregnancy anyway. If you bleed, you will need an urgent INR.

Patients on life-long warfarin for clots in the lungs

If you are on life-long warfarin for proven severe blood clots in your lungs (pulmonary emboli causing chronic thromboembolic disease associated pulmonary hypertension) you must be very careful indeed about your warfarin. This is the most important part of all your treatments.

You will need to convert to clexane injections in your skin if you need to stop your warfarin temporarily for any reason (e.g. a heart catheter test).

Oxygen

How does it work?

Most patients with PAH have a slightly low level of oxygen in their blood which would not make them breathless. Oxygen treatment does not help breathlessness unless the oxygen level is very low. This is measured with an oximeter. A level under 90% might make you breathless. Tests are done in the lung function department to help us decide which patients will benefit from oxygen treatment. Your PAH team will tell you if you need oxygen or not.

 Most PAH patients do not benefit from oxygen and so do not need it.

In patients with severe lung disease, arteries in areas of the lung with a low oxygen level clamp down, and this is another cause of high lung artery pressures. Oxygen treatment opens up these arteries, lowers the lung artery pressure, and improves the blood supply to these parts of the lungs. Therefore oxygen treatment should be given to patients where low oxygen levels are the cause of high pressure in the lungs. This improves their survival and ability to exercise.

What you need to do

We advise patients who benefit from oxygen to take 16 hours of oxygen per day and during physical activity. They should take oxygen throughout the day and night if they are unwell or have a chest infection. A *fitness to fly test* will tell us if they need oxygen during an air flight.

Oxygen is available on the NHS. The PAH team and PAH-UK will advise you on how to get it. Oxygen is stored in cylinders supplied by a local pharmacy and delivered to your home together with a mask. Alternatively, small plastic tubes called nasal cannulae are put in the nostrils. This leaves the mouth clear and allows you to eat, drink, and talk without taking the mask off. Oxygen flowing in the nasal tubes can dry out the nose. Your PAH team will give you advice on how to use ointments to prevent crusting and damage to the inside of your nose. If you take oxygen you must not smoke, and you should certainly not smoke while breathing oxygen or you might cause a fire or an explosion.

Oxygen can also be obtained from an oxygen concentrator machine. This is the size of a small refrigerator and extracts oxygen from the air. This is the most convenient method for people on oxygen throughout the day. A back-up oxygen cylinder should also be available. An engineer will install and maintain the oxygen concentrator for you, and they are easy to use.

Your GP should be able to get for you semi-portable oxygen cylinders which deliver a set rate of oxygen. There is also a system (flow regulator or conserver) which pumps oxygen through the tubes only when you breathe in. This prevents wastage of oxygen compared with a continuous flow system.

Very good, small, and light oxygen cylinders have recently become available for people to use when they go out for a couple of hours shopping or for other activities.

Digoxin

What it does

Digoxin in its natural form (the foxglove) has been in use as a herbal remedy for dropsy (heart failure) for hundreds of years. The first recorded use of foxglove powder as a poison goes back to the Persian Empire.

Digoxin improves symptoms without either improving or worsening survival. In PAH it helps the right heart beat more strongly, and by slowing the heart allows it to fill with blood more easily. However, digoxin is very dangerous if too much is taken, and doses must be kept very low especially if your kidneys are not working well. Digoxin has been studied fully in patients with left heart failure, and is used in PAH based on experience and short-term studies in right heart failure.

Occasionally, some patients develop an irregular heart rhythm called atrial fibrillation. Digoxin slows the heart rate down and helps the heart beat more efficiently.

What you have to do

In the dose commonly used (0.125 mg per day) digoxin rarely causes side-effects. It does not interact with any of the other drugs commonly used to treat PAH. It can be taken together with all your other tablets at any time of the day, before or after meals.

12

Targeted therapy

🡒 Key points

♦ In PAH there are faults in the cells lining the lung arteries (endothelium), which either cannot produce the chemicals needed to keep the lung arteries healthy or produce too many harmful chemicals. At least three key chemicals are lacking. There are three groups or families of drugs which restore these chemicals to more normal levels. Two are given as tablets. The third is given into a vein or into the skin.

♦ The two groups of tablets are endothelin receptor antagonists (ERAs) and phosphodiesterase-5 (PDE-5) inhibitors. ERAs (drugs with names ending in '…tan') reduce the thickening in the lung artery walls to allow more blood to flow through the lungs.

♦ Phosphodiesterase-5 (PDE-5) inhibitors (drugs with names ending in '… fil') relax and widen the lung arteries and improve the blood flow through the lungs.

♦ The third group of drugs are called prostanoids. Prostanoids are synthetic (man-made) drugs similar to the naturally produced substance prostacyclin. They are given into the vein, through the skin, or by inhalation.

♦ All these drugs lower the pressure in the lung arteries, make patients feel better, and allow them to walk slightly further. They slow down the progression of the disease. Because no 'head-to-head' trials comparing these drugs have been done, we do not know if one group is better than the others, or if one member of a group is better than the other members of the same group. Until we know, we assume that all members within a group are similar.

♦ New drugs are being developed. We hope that quality of life and survival for our patients will continue to improve.

Groups of drugs that 'target' abnormalities in lung arteries

There are three groups of drugs which reduce lung artery wall thickening. They are called *disease-modifying treatments*:

- prostanoids (man-made chemicals which have the same effects as prostacyclin)
- endothelin receptor antagonists (ERAs)
- phosphodiesterase-5 (PDE-5) inhibitors

In clinical trials, each of these groups of drugs:

- improves symptoms
- improves exercise capacity
- improves quality of life
- reduces the pressure in the lung arteries
- increases blood flow through the lungs
- slows down the disease.

The prostanoids

- **Prostaglandins** are a group of chemicals produced by endothelial cells in blood vessels of different organs. They relax and widen blood vessels, they help to control things like childbirth, they aid wound repair, and they reduce blood clotting. Prostaglandin E was shown to relax lung vessels 30 years ago, and so it was thought that it might be useful in PAH.

- **Prostacyclin** is a naturally produced chemical messenger and is member of the prostaglandin group of chemicals. Prostacyclin relaxes and widens all arteries, partially stops blood clotting, and stops the lining cells of the lung arteries from growing and multiplying.

- **Prostanoids** are man-made forms of prostacyclin.

PAH patients do not make enough prostacyclin. Giving prostanoids 'tops up' the low level of prostacyclin. There are several different types of prostanoid which all have similar effects.

Prostanoids were the first effective treatments for PAH. They improve survival, symptoms, and exercise capacity, and reduce the heart and lung artery pressures. They are effective even in the sickest patients, and they work long term. There is no evidence that one prostanoid is better than the others; however, only epoprostanol has been tested in the sickest people with pulmonary hypertension. The choice of prostanoid is tailored to the patient and the patient's preference.

Prostanoids are usually reserved for patients who have not responded to or cannot tolerate other forms of treatment (ERAs and PDE-5 inhibitors), and patients with severe PAH.

How prostanoids work

All prostanoids work in the same way. When prostanoids were first used in PAH it was hoped that, as with ordinary blood pressure medications, they would reduce the blood pressure to normal, but they did not. People continued using them because patients felt better even though the pressure in the lung vessels stayed much the same. With prolonged use of prostanoids, the lung pressures seemed to fall more than they did in the first few minutes of use, although the fall in pressure is only slight. It is now thought that prostanoids work by attacking the main problem in PAH—they suppress the growth of cells within the lung artery walls.

Side-effects of prostanoids

Side-effects with prostanoids can be quite troublesome. Therefore the starting dose is low and gradually increased to let the body get used to the drug. The side-effects are jaw pain, headache, feeling hot and sweaty, nausea, and diarrhoea and vomiting. These side-effects usually disappear after a while and most patients get used to them. Occasionally, if the side-effects are bad, the dose may have to be reduced. Because the majority of patients on prostanoids have severe PAH and may have already tried other treatments, it is important for patients to be aware of these side-effects and not give up on the drug too quickly.

Epoprostanol (Flolan)

Epoprostanol is a synthetic prostacyclin. It is a freeze-dried powder which is dissolved in water for infusion. It is pumped by a small battery-powered pump worn in a pouch around the waist through a very thin plastic tube (Hickman line) which is tunnelled under the skin on the front of the chest into a large vein under the collar bone.

Epoprostenol is an unstable chemical and lasts for only a few minutes in blood before it changes and becomes inactive. That is why it has to be continuously pumped into the body. This is a drawback because of the small but important risk of infection getting into the body from the line. If the line becomes infected, the infection may spread to the heart and then all around the body. However, the risk of this happening is very low because the line is put in with scrupulous care, under sterile conditions, by a specialist in an operating room or cardiac catheter laboratory. X rays are used to make sure that the end of the line is in the right position in the superior vena cava. Once the line is in, it is essential that the patient and, if necessary, a family member, know how to keep it clean, make up the solution of drug to the correct dose, which is periodically increased, and know how to work the pump and what to do if things go wrong. Patients are admitted to hospital so that the PAH specialist nurses can train them to make sure that they are completely competent and confident about all aspects of the system. It is not difficult, and virtually all patients learn how to use the system without any problem. The pump reservoir has to be changed every 12 hours.

If the line does become infected, it usually has to be removed immediately to avoid the risk of infection spreading to the heart and the rest of the body (septicaemia). Sometimes, the infection is mild and responds to antibiotics.

Trepostinil (Remodulin or UT-15)

The other commonly used prostanoid is called trepostinil. There is no evidence that it is better or worse than epoprostenol. It is man-made, more stable than epoprostenol, and lasts longer in the blood stream (3 hours compared with a few minutes for epoprostenol).

Trepostinil comes as a ready-to-use fluid and so is easier to set up than epoprostenol. Patients are admitted to hospital for a few days to learn how to use the system. Trepostinil is drawn up by a syringe which is inserted into a very small pump which is put into a pouch and strapped around the waist. The trepostinil is then pumped through very thin plastic tubing into the skin of the tummy through a tiny needle. The line, pump, and skin must be kept clean to avoid the risk of infection. The reservoir in the pump needs to be refilled every 48 hours.

The dose is increased from time to time depending on the patient's response and whether they have side-effects. The common side-effects are temporary reddening, thickening, and tenderness of the skin where the needle is inserted. Anaesthetic creams are used, but these are not completely effective. The needle is moved to different sites every few days because the drug may not be absorbed if the skin becomes hard. The skin hardening and tenderness usually resolve after a few days.

Over 70% of patients find this system acceptable. Those who do not may be switched to intravenous prostanoids.

Recently treprostinil has also been shown to be effective when inhaled through a nebulizer, and will soon be available in this form. This has the advantage that, with a relatively long-lived prostanoid like treprostinil, only four inhalations per day are required.

Iloprost (Ventavis)

Iloprost is a synthetic liquid prostanoid. It is given through a mask from a machine called a nebulizer, which converts the fluid to a spray. It does not take long for patients to learn how to set up the machine.

Each inhalation takes around 10 minutes to complete. The effects last for a couple of hours and so at least six doses have to be taken each day, starting as soon as you wake up. Patients may find the necessity for frequent inhalations a major inconvenience because they disrupt their daily activities.

Beraprost

This is a tablet form of prostanoid which does not appear to offer any advantage over other prostanoids and has not been shown to exert long-term benefits. As a result this form is not licensed except in Japan.

Endothelin receptor antagonists

Endothelin is a chemical made by the cells lining artery walls (endothelium) in all parts of the body. Endothelin makes arteries constrict and narrow. Patients with PAH have too much endothelin in their lung arteries, and this is a problem as it causes constriction of lung arteries, an increase in the size and number of cells in the artery walls, and overgrowth and narrowing of the artery.

How ERAs work

Endothelin, in common with many other chemical messengers, works by attaching itself to a protein or receptor on a cell, a bit like a boat hooking up to a mooring post. Once attached to a receptor, there is a sequence of chemical reactions in the cell resulting in a variety of changes depending on which cells and which molecules are 'turned on'. In PAH, the arteries become thicker and narrower.

Once endothelin was discovered and its actions understood, chemicals were developed to block its attachment to receptors so that it could not work. These chemicals blocking, or antagonizing, its attachment to its receptors are called endothelin receptor antagonists (ERAs). The bad effects of endothelin are blocked.

The first ERA was bosentan (Tracleer) and there are now two others, sitaxentan (Thelin) and ambrisentan (Volibris). Other similar ERAs are in development. There is no evidence that one ERA is better than the others. Trials have been conducted with all ERAs, but not over long periods of time.

What have ERAs been shown to do?

All three ERAs:

- are tablets taken once or twice a day
- help in various types of PAH
- may upset the liver in a minority of patients
- improve exercise capacity
- improve functional class
- lower lung artery pressures
- slow down progression of the disease.

Side-effects of ERAs

Because ERAs upset the liver in around 5–10% of patients, they are not usually given to patients with liver disease. They can also lower the haemoglobin (blood count). It is essential to have monthly blood tests for liver function and full blood count. The PAH team will help you arrange this near your home. If the liver function tests become very abnormal, the ERA should be stopped. It may take several weeks for the liver function to return to normal (it virtually always does) and then either a different ERA or another type of drug can be tried.

Other side-effects include puffy feet and legs, stuffy nose, flushing, palpitations, tummy ache, and constipation.

Women of child-bearing age who have PAH are advised not to become pregnant because of the near 50% risk of death. Women of child-bearing age taking ERAs should also have a monthly pregnancy test.

Quite often a patient who cannot tolerate one ERA can tolerate a different one. ERAs may affect the quality of sperm.

Interactions of ERAs with other tablets are listed in Table 12.1.

Table 12.1 Drug interactions of ERAs

ERA	Drug interaction
Ambrisentan	Levels of ciclosporin and ketoconazole are reduced and so larger doses of these drugs may be necessary.
Bosentan	Sildenafil levels fall by 50%. Bosentan levels increase by 50%. However, dose adjustments may not be necessary.
	Ciclosporin levels fall by 50%. Bosentan levels increase fourfold. Ciclosporin should not be given to patients on bosentan.
	Erythromycin increase bosentan levels.
	Ketoconazole increases bosentan levels.
	Glibenclamide effects are reduced and so sugar levels rise.
	Amiodarone increases bosentan level.
	Phenytoin and rifampicin lower bosentan level by 50%.
	Statin levels reduced by 50%.
	Warfarin level reduced. Warfarin dose may need to be increased.
	Oral contraceptive level reduced with increased pregnancy risk.
Sitaxentan	Warfarin dose always needs to be reduced because of decreased metabolism of warfarin.
	Ciclosporin increases sitaxentan level. Should not be used with sitaxentan.

Dosages of ERAs

◆ Bosentan (Tracleer) is started at 62.5 mg twice a day and increased to 125 mg twice a day after 4 weeks if there are no side-effects.

◆ Sitaxentan (Thelin) is started and continued at 100 mg once a day.

◆ Ambrisentan (Volibris) is started at 5 mg a day and, if there are no side-effects, increased after 4 weeks to 10 mg a day.

Phosphodiesterase-5 inhibitors (PDE-5 inhibitors)

These drugs became famous in the form of Viagra, which is used for impotence. Sildenafil (Viagra) and tadalafil (Cialis) open up arteries and improve the blood supply to the penis. For impotence, one tablet is taken about an hour before intercourse.

In PAH, three tablets of Sildenafil are taken a day long term to help keep the lung arteries open. For reasons which are not clear, when used in this fashion they have no sexual effect. This may be because the psychology of taking treatment for PAH is very different from taking a tablet to help impotence.

PDE-5 inhibitors are generally safe and well tolerated, and can be taken with most other tablets and medications. They can be taken either before or after meals.

How PDE-5 inhibitors work in PAH

PDE-5 inhibitors prevent the action of the enzyme (phosphodiesterase) which destroys nitric oxide, a naturally occurring chemical produced by the endothelium. Nitric oxide is a powerful vasodilator which relaxes and opens arteries, allowing more blood and oxygen to flow to the lung. This is why it works in impotence (erectile dysfunction).

As well as improving the blood supply to the lung by dilating lung arteries, which may be in spasm or constricted, PDE-5 inhibitors also reduce the overgrowth and number of cells in the artery wall.

What have PDE-5 inhibitors been shown to do?

PDE-5 inhibitors can be used in all types of PAH. They improve symptoms and exercise performance, and slow down the progression of the disease.

Side-effects of PDE-5 inhibitors

These are uncommon and not usually severe or troublesome. They are related to the way that the drugs work by opening up arteries. Headache, feeling flushed, and nose bleeds may occur. Some people on other PAH medication have a low blood pressure, and their blood pressure may fall a bit more if a PDE-5 inhibitor is added. Before starting on sildenafil, the blood pressure is taken and checked after taking a test tablet to make sure that it does not fall too much. Drug interactions are listed in Table 12.2.

Table 12.2 Drug interactions of PDE-5 inhibitors

PDE-5 inhibitor	Interaction
Sildenafil	GTN, nitrates, or nicorandil taken with sildenafil may cause low blood pressure. Sildenafil and nitrates cannot be taken together.
	Bosentan lowers sildenafil levels by 50%. Bosentan levels increase by 50%. However, dose adjustments may not be necessary.
	Statin levels may increase. Sildenafil levels may increase.
	HIV drugs increase the level of sildenafil and so the sildenafil dose may need to be reduced.
	Phenytoin may reduce the levels of sildenafil.
	Erythromycin increases the sildenafil level. If erythromycin is used for only a few days, no dose adjustment of sildenafil is necessary.
	Ketoconazole increases the level of sildenafil but it is not necessary to change the dose of either drug.
	Rifampicin reduces the availability of sildenafil to almost nothing.
Tadalafil	GTN, nitrates, or nicorandil taken with tadalafil may cause severe low blood pressure. Tadalafil and nitrates cannot be taken together.
	Bosentan lowers tadalafil levels by 40%. Bosentan levels remain the same. No need to change dosages of either tablet.

GTN, glyceryl trinitrate

Calcium-channel blockers (nifedipine, diltiazem, amlodipine)

These are used to treat idiopathic PAH (IPAH) and familial PAH (FPAH) in patients who have a positive vasodilator response at the time of right heart catheterization. A positive vasodilator response is defined as a lowering of the mean lung pressure by at least 10 mmHg to less than 40 mmHg. Calcium-channel blockers are not used in other forms of PAH.

Unfortunately, only a small proportion (10%) of patients with IPAH have a positive vasodilator response at the time of right heart catheterization. Only 50% of these responding patients have a sustained response to calcium-channel blockers. Therefore, calcium-channel blockers are likely to benefit only 5% of patients with IPAH long term.

How calcium-channel blockers work in PAH

Calcium-channel blockers relax and widen constricted lung arteries, improving the blood supply to the lungs.

What have calcium-channel blockers been shown to do?

In a minority of patients with IPAH or FPAH, they can lower the lung pressures to normal or very close to normal. This small proportion of patients feel very much better and lead a normal or near-normal life. It is not known how long this response lasts.

Side-effects

The common side-effects with nifedipine and amlodipine are foot and ankle swelling and feeling flushed. The fluid accumulation in the legs can be treated with water tablets (diuretics).

Calcium-channel blockers are commonly used to treat systemic (ordinary) high blood pressure. Most PAH patients have normal blood pressure. Therefore PAH patients taking calcium-channel blockers may have a low blood pressure and feel light-headed or faint. One type of calcium-channel blocker, diltiazem, can slow the heart rate quite considerably as well as lowering the blood pressure.

Doses of calcium-channel blockers

- Nifedipine 120–240 mg a day
- Diltiazem 240–720 mg a day
- Amlodipine 20 mg a day

These doses are much higher than those used to treat systemic hypertension and that is why PAH patients may feel light headed on these doses. The dose can be lowered, but this may reduce the effect of the calcium-channel blocker on the PAH.

Guidelines and choosing medications for patients

Each PAH specialist has their own preferred approach to treating PAH. Some may prefer to use a PDE-5 inhibitor first and then an ERA. Some prefer an ERA as first-line treatment. Some prefer one ERA over another. Others may prefer to use prostanoids and have a preference for one particular prostanoid. This is perfectly understandable if there is not compelling evidence to choose one medication over the others, except in certain cases.

New drugs, new members of each group of drugs, and the results of new clinical trials make the treatment of PAH exciting and optimistic for PAH specialists and patients, but also confusing. There is no single 'correct' way to treat a patient. Each patient is unique in every respect.

Practice guidelines provide clinicians with a framework for clinical management based on the best available evidence from trials judged by a consensus of experts. Guidelines are not law. They are a map, and clinicians use the map to plan a route for their patients based on the guidelines. However, several routes can be taken. It is quite common to use one tablet and then for various reasons, including inadequate response or intolerability, to change to a different medication. PAH patients are carefully and closely monitored to make sure that they remain on the right road.

Which drug to use first?

Generally, tablets are used first because they are easier to take. PAH clinicians use drugs that they are used to and with which they are most familiar.

◆ For patients in WHO class 2, ambrisentan, bosentan, sildenafil or tadalafil could be used.

◆ For patients in WHO class 3, ambrisentan, bosentan, sitaxentan, sildenafil, epoprostenol, inhaled iloprost, tadalafil, or subcutaneous or inhaled trepostinil could be used.

◆ Because prostanoids are given into a vein or into the skin, they are generally reserved for patients with severe PAH who tend to have already been treated with tablets.

◆ Prostanoids are used as a first-line treatment if patients are first diagnosed at this severe stage (WHO class 4).

Some patients, who are first diagnosed when they are in WHO class 4, might not want to start with a prostanoid. Under these circumstances, they could be treated with a tablet or a combination of an ERA and PDE-5 inhibitor combined together as 'initial combination therapy'. If this approach does not work after a month or so and the patient is deteriorating, they should be treated with a prostanoid and one or both tablets gradually reduced and stopped if possible.

Combination therapy

Although it is not clear whether combining different types of PAH treatments to be taken together is more effective and safe in the long term, it makes sense. There are at least three different problems causing PAH and so treating all of them, or at least two of them, at once is appealing.

At the moment, we do not know the best combination of drugs, or when the drugs should be combined (early on or only after one has been shown to be inadequate). There is evidence from trials that combinations of prostanoids with both PDE-5 inhibitors and ERAs, and ERAs with PDE-5 inhibitors, are effective. So far the most powerful combination appears to be epoprostenol and sildenafil.

Rewriting guidelines

Guidelines need to rewritten as soon as they become out of date based on new evidence from trials.

13

When medication is not enough

➲ Key points

- Lung transplantation and atrial septostomy are offered to patients with end-stage PAH.

- Lungs or heart and lungs can be transplanted. The shortage of both organs restricts these treatments to only a few patients.

- There are significant risks of infection and rejection after lung transplantation.

- Atrial septostomy is a procedure done in the cardiac catheter laboratory. A hole is made in the partition wall separating the two atria (collecting chambers). This reduces the pressure in the right heart but reduces the oxygen level further by diverting blood away from the lungs to the left side of the heart. It can be of help in young patients with congenital heart disease while they await heart and lung transplantation. It is not clear when it should be performed to provide the most benefit.

- Thrombo-endarterectomy—removal of blood clots from lung arteries blocked by blood clots—can help some patients, but there are considerable risks. Patients need to continue on PAH medications after surgery, which is done in only one centre in the UK.

Lung transplantation

Lung transplantation is an extreme form of treatment, but very logical. The problem in PAH is in the lung vessels. Because it is not possible to change or transplant individual lung arteries, a whole lung or both lungs have to be replaced. If the right heart has failed and is not likely to recover, the heart should also be replaced. This is a major operation and patients have to be fit enough to have it. One in five people die within 30 days. Powerful drugs are needed to prevent rejection of the transplanted lungs and heart. Over the years the treatments on the body's immune systems take their toll; new lungs become damaged within 5 years.

The results of lung transplantation are not nearly as good as kidney, liver, or heart transplants, because of rejection and lung failure. Some lung transplant patients survive for 10 years or more with a good quality of life, while other patients live for only a few months or less. Only half the patients survive for 5 years.

Certain conditions, including poorly controlled diabetes and related complications in other organs, severe mental health problems, significant coronary artery disease, severe reflux of acid from the stomach due to scleroderma, and cancer (other than localized skin cancers), make a patient unsuitable for transplantation.

Support from family or friends is essential for a successful outcome because of the complicated post-transplant care.

Even with all these problems it is still quite an attractive option, but until the problems of donor numbers and rejection are solved it will remain an exceptional treatment.

Patients who are suitable may be referred to a transplant centre if they do not respond fairly quickly to a prostanoid. They meet the transplant team on several occasions when all aspects of the operation are explained.

Atrial septostomy

This is rarely done in the UK. It is considered as a last ditch attempt to help patients who have deteriorated despite combination therapy. Some are awaiting or being considered for transplantation.

It is a relatively simple operation that can be done at the same time as cardiac catheterization. A small hole is punched between the right and left filling chambers of the heart (atria). This allows blood to bypass the lungs completely. More blood circulates to the left heart and although this reduces the work the right heart has to do, the left heart has more work to do. In the short term, this is not a major problem. The blood bypassing the lungs does not pick up any oxygen and so patients become blue (cyanosed).

This procedure is very effective in young children as it stops them blacking out. In older people there is a greater risk of stroke as blood travelling from right to left can carry clots with it, and the procedure itself is moderately hazardous. If the hole made in the atrial partition wall (atrial septum) is too big, the body is starved of oxygen because none circulates to the lungs.

Some people benefit and some are made worse. Atrial septostomy does nothing to correct the underlying problem in PAH, which continues to progress. Nevertheless, it may be of short term benefit for patients who are very sick and whose right heart is very weak. Patients have to be fit enough to be considered for the procedure. It has not really caught on as a treatment except in countries where effective drugs are not available.

Thrombo-endarterectomy

It is very important to see if a breathless patient has blood clots in the lungs. If they do, this can explain their symptoms. The most important part of their treatment is blood thinning (anticoagulation) with warfarin, or a similar drug, for at least 6 months. PAH patients are generally advised to take warfarin for life to reduce the risk of clots even if they have not had any. Those whose PAH is due to clots in the lungs should certainly be on anticoagulants. Patients on warfarin need regular blood tests (usually every 6–8 weeks) to make sure that their dose of warfarin is correct.

Only one centre in the UK, Papworth Hospital, does this operation. Even though it is risky, if done in carefully selected patients, the results are very good and previously very breathless patients can return to normal or near-normal physical activities.

End-of-life issues and terminal care

Unfortunately, death comes to us all. PAH, like many other diseases, is managed with medicines rather than cured by therapy. Although the outlook is now vastly improved compared with the situation just a few years ago, and more improvements are expected over the next few years, the reality is that true stability is not yet achieved in enough patients. With current therapies most patients improve and have a much better quality of life for the first couple of years on treatment. With changes and increases in the number of treatments used, even those with very resistant progressive disease usually respond, at least initially. For those whose condition is stable for around 4 years, the condition often enters a period of prolonged stability.

However, there are those for whom the therapies are not strong enough to stop the disease worsening. These patients usually become more breathless because of the increasing lung artery pressures putting a strain on the right heart. Most of these patients know what is going on and understand that their condition is no longer responding to treatment. They know that they are coming to the end of the road. Despite their problems, they are usually remarkably calm about the prospect of dying, but are concerned for their family and about the possibility of their suffering continuing. One major worry is how to discuss these issues with their family and their carers.

The great advantage of PAH specialist centres is that the PAH team get to know their patients very well. We encourage open and frank discussions when medical treatment begins to fail and a patient deteriorates. Patients and the PAH team need to feel able to discuss the end-stage of treatment without fear or reluctance. It is important to remember that, with the medicines now available, no one needs to die in a state of distress or suffer unpleasant breathlessness, and other symptoms can almost always be managed.

Some patients prefer and are able to be looked after at home. Others prefer to be admitted to a hospice. Pain control, relief of anxiety, fluids and nutrition, and psychological and, where wanted, spiritual support are essential and will be offered to all patients. In the UK, the Macmillan team offer unrivalled expertise and care and should be contacted for patients who would like palliative care.

14

Living your life

General principles for keeping fit, strong, and healthy

These guidelines and suggestions are not based on scientific evidence, just common sense and our experience of dealing with many patients with all types of PAH and other medical conditions. With treatment, most patients have a reasonable or excellent quality of life, and many can continue to work. However, as with any serious condition, the psychological impact of the disease can be very debilitating.

 Case history

Susan was 22 when she noticed that her hands became cold and went white, even in summer. She was told that she had Raynaud's disease. When she was in her late forties, the skin of her hands and feet became stiff, thickened, and tight. A rheumatologist told her that she now had scleroderma. Because around 12% of scleroderma patients develop PAH, she was screened for PAH every year with an echocardiogram and lung function tests. Over the next few years she gradually became tired and breathless doing the housework and walking up hills. The test results also became abnormal.

She was referred to the PAH specialists who advised her to have a right heart catheter test. This showed that she had PAH. She was devastated. Her husband gave up his job to be with her. She was treated with an ERA, and then sildenafil was added because her lung artery pressure remained high.

Over the next few months, she began to feel less breathless. Her heart pressures and lung pressures improved. Her six-minute walk distance stabilized in the high 300 metre range.

But despite these bits of good news, she felt terrible. She had lost her confidence, spending most of the day at home with her wonderfully supportive husband, crying and feeling petrified. She lost her ability to think about what she was able to do; she did not feel able to walk down to the sea front, to go out for lunch, or to be with friends and family. Her fear of herself, the diagnosis of PAH, and her total lack of self-confidence were now her main immediate problems. Her breathing remained quite good.

She looked well and always put on a brave face when she and her husband came to the joint PAH and scleroderma clinic. But during one consultation, when she was reassured and told that again her six-minute walk test and blood tests were stable, Susan and her husband broke down and cried. Only then did they tell the PAH team about the way they felt. Managing complex cases of PAH demands more than just 'doing the tests, prescribing and arranging medication, and saying goodbye'. The clinicians and the patient and their family 'are in it together'. Unless the clinicians ask the right questions, and the patients say how they feel and what really concerns them, essential aspects will not be addressed.

A plan was hatched and agreed. Susan and her husband live 60 miles from her PAH centre. Susan phones the PAH specialist nurses every week to tell them what she has done that week, focusing on the good days and the enjoyable aspects of the week. She tells them her plans for the next week. She is encouraged to keep going and continue with the social activities she likes to do. In addition Susan is encouraged to exercise every day, walking at her own pace (including resting whenever necessary) for at least 10 minutes per day.

Slowly, Susan has returned to a near-normal life. Her breathing and energy levels are not great, but she leads a quiet but much more active life and gets out and about. She does something nice every day. She and her husband go out for lunch once or twice a week. She invites friends round for a cup of tea. She and her husband go away for long weekends. Susan plucked up courage and enjoyed a short cruise. With support and encouragement and some direct talking from the PAH team, she was able to escape from her self-imposed prison. She found the key to the world outside and had the courage to keep going.

Lessons from the case history

It is essential for PAH patients to try to be as positive as possible about life every day, even if the condition limits daily activity. Of course this is simplistic and easy to say. But the opposite is defeatist and giving up is unhelpful to you.

Try to see the sun through the clouds. Look for the rainbow of hope and remain optimistic. This attitude, coupled with excellent medical and nursing care, and strong support from friends and family, will provide extra energy to help you through any bad days you have. Being positive will make it easier for your supporters to support you, and there are always people there on your side.

Ultimately, it is up to you. It is a daunting prospect, but the human spirit is unbelievably strong and formidable, and this has been shown over and over again during the past during all sorts of terrible human disasters.

Mental and physical strength

Possibly the most important thing you can do to help yourself is to keep psychologically and physically strong. This is easier with support and encouragement from family and friends. Your PAH team—doctors, nurses, pharmacists, physiotherapists, and other specialized staff—are all there to help, guide, and advise you and your family. They can answer your questions and concerns and, where possible, allay your anxieties and fears.

You should:

* maintain a positive attitude, be confident and optimistic, and not lose your sense of humour
* do something enjoyable every day
* keep active with some daily exercise
* eat a healthy balanced diet
* rest when you feel like it and sleep well
* make life easy for yourself
* surround yourself with nice supportive positive people.

> Keep going. Never give up. Never let your head drop. Never lose your hope and optimism.

Exercise: how often and how much?

All patients should try to do some form of physical exercise or movement every day. This applies even to patients who become breathless with minimal exertion. For most patients walking is the most important exercise. The six-minute walk test gives us a rough idea of how much exercise you should aim for: those managing over 500 metres in 6 minutes should be able to walk fairly normally; most of those managing 350–500 metres should be able to walk at their own pace on the level for 10 minutes; those managing less than 350 metres often need to rest after walking a short distance, get their breath, and walk the same distance again. The most important thing when exercising is not to push it so hard that you are in danger of blacking out (feeling faint), or do so much that you feel completely exhausted and would not wish to do the same next day.

The level of activity you will be able to manage depends on several factors: your age, the severity of your PAH, the state of your heart and lungs, the presence of other medical conditions affecting your skin, muscles, and joints, your previous physical condition, and whether you were sporty and fit when you were younger. The key thing is your mental attitude.

We encourage all PAH patients to do whatever they can to remain supple, toned, strong, and flexible. You should exercise and stretch your arm and leg muscles as often as you can during the day. The more exercise you do, the more you will be able to do. Sitting or lying down for long periods makes you weak and stiff. It is also depressing.

You should try to lead a full and active life every day. Unless you are breathless at rest, doing nothing, it is generally safe for you to push yourself a little until you feel breathless. Stop if you feel very breathless or light-headed and think you might faint.

Every patient knows their limits. You will know if you are overdoing things; you will feel breathless and exhausted. It is safe for you to get slightly breathless and tired. Stop and rest if you feel light-headed or very breathless, or if your heart beats uncomfortably fast.

> Most PAH patients are better and fitter than they think they. It is safe to exercise, move your arms and legs, and feel slightly breathless and exhausted. You will know if you are overdoing things. If you have to stop—stop and rest.

Exercise and functional class

The intensity of exercise that a patient can do depends on their functional class—the level of activities they can do comfortably.

WHO class 1 patients

These patients have PAH but can lead a normal life without breathlessness or exercise limitations. They lead a full and active life and can walk long distances up and down hills, do housework and gardening, and even play sports and go to the gym. Their friends and family may not even notice that there is something wrong with them.

WHO class 4 patients

At the other end of the spectrum are patients with severe PAH who are breathless at rest. They may need oxygen throughout the day or if they do even slight exercise. Some may be restricted to a wheelchair. They may not be able to do much for themselves.

Gentle slow arm and leg movements can be done in a high-backed chair. This keeps the circulation going and helps maintain tone in the arm and leg muscles.

WHO class 2 and 3 patients

The majority of PAH patients are in between these two groups of patients. Many are at least reasonably comfortable doing moderate or gentle exercise, but may feel breathless and exhausted if they overdo things and walk too fast or go up stairs or hills.

> On a good day, be as active as you can. On a bad day, take it easy and rest. Play it by ear.

Ten general principles for living with PAH

1. Think positive thoughts, keep your spirits up, and concentrate on what is good in your life. Count your blessings. You have plenty, but may not always be able to see them because you are focusing on the bad things about your life. As soon as you start to feel morose, depressed, and tearful, and things seem hopeless, think of the good things you have: your family and friends, good memories, your achievements, the ability to see, hear, and think, and the ability to continue to experience and enjoy nice things. Life is rarely absolutely awful. It is the way that you see things at the time.

2. If you work and want to continue to work, think of ways that your daily work and travel programme can be made easier for you, and then try to arrange this. Your GP and the PHA-UK organization may be able to provide practical help and advice.

3. Try to do something enjoyable and fun every day—something that will make you smile and make you feel content. Plan as much of your week as you can in advance.

4. Don't over do things and don't overfill your diary. Rest when you have to and even when you don't think you need to. If you get tired during the day, live the Mediterranean life. Take a siesta, a snooze, or 40 winks every day after lunch. Regular good-quality sleep at night is important.

5. Surround yourself with as many nice, supportive, and helpful people as you can. Try to cheer others up—this will help you. There are many others much worse off than you. Tea parties, going out for a meal or a film, and visiting friends, family, and neighbours are all part of normal relationships. Keep them going.

6. If you are in pain or very distressed, speak to your PAH team, your PAH patient organization, or your GP for practical help and support.

7. If you can get away for a change of scene for a night or two, or an even longer break somewhere, try to go. It may be a daunting thought, but even very sick people can go away with careful planning and this can be a terrific boost.

8. Make your life as comfortable and easy as you can. Think through your daily schedule or timetable with your friends and family. Your GP may be able to arrange for an occupational therapist or social worker to help you with your daily activities (cleaning, cooking, bathing, and shopping).

9. Increase your leisure activities (music, reading, radio, listening books, TV, entertainments, and anything else you enjoy).

10. PHA-UK and religious organizations are usually very supportive and helpful.

♦ You are a member of a large supportive, sympathetic, helpful, and under-standing community of patients, their families, and a strong committed team of experts from a variety of clinical backgrounds who are there and available to help.

♦ You are not alone.

♦ Go to bed with the positive warm thought: 'That was a good day, and I enjoyed it. I wonder what good things tomorrow will bring?' Smile when you think of the good days. Accept the bad days, knowing that the next day will be good. After the rain, comes the sun.

♦ Wake up thinking 'I am alive and kicking. What enjoyable, worthwhile things am I going to do today?' Do them.

Food and drink

Eat what you like, when you like

The majority of PAH patients can eat and drink more or less whatever they want. Eat when you are hungry.

There are no 'superfoods'

There is no evidence that certain foods or drink make PAH worse, and no evidence that certain foods or drink make it better. There is no evidence that vitamin supplements, herbal remedies, organic foods, or other 'wonder foods' marketed by food manufacturers affect the condition one way or the other. If you like certain foods, eat them and enjoy them.

The important principle is to eat a full and healthy diet, with a balance of protein (meats, eggs, fish), carbohydrate (potatoes, bread, pizza, pasta, rice), and dairy foods (for calcium and other vitamins). A full range of vegetables, fruit, and salad will give you all the vitamins and minerals you need. Unless you cannot or do not eat a balanced diet, there is no need for you to take vitamin supplements. Drink plenty of water if you are thirsty. If you are a vegetarian, try to eat as broad a range of healthy foods as you can to make sure that you are not excluding essential vitamins and minerals.

It is important to maintain your required calorie intake. Being overweight or too thin are both bad.

Maintain you fuel and calorie intake

In contrast to the dietary advice we give obese or overweight people who have systemic hypertension, heart problems, diabetes, and a high cholesterol level, patients with severe PAH are often underweight and have a poor appetite. They tend not to have a high cholesterol level or systemic hypertension, but if they do, we advise them to eat a balanced healthy diet and achieve an optimum weight. A minority of PAH patients have diabetes and a high cholesterol level, but these conditions are easy to treat.

Thin people who have a poor appetite or difficulty in swallowing or absorbing food should have a high-calorie diet: carbohydrates (bread, pasta, rice, potatoes) and fat (dairy foods, cheese, butter, chocolate, cakes, biscuits, deserts). Some patients cannot tolerate or do not like these high-calorie foods. There are a variety of high-calorie drinks, including Ensure and other similar 'complete' drinks, which are high in calories and also contain vitamins and minerals. One or two glasses of these drinks a day are helpful in maintaining weight and are a good source of energy. Your GP can prescribe these for you.

Obesity is rare in PAH. Overweight patients should try to eat a low-calorie diet to achieve their optimum target weight.

Mealtimes

These are important times of the day when you can sit down and be with your family and friends. Mealtimes provide a formal structure and rhythm to your day. Unless eating is a really difficult or embarrassing problem, try to eat with people and try to enjoy your food. It is an important part of life. If you find cooking and preparing meals difficult, or you just don't enjoy doing it, ask a family member or friend to help you.

Preparing your food

Unless you are really very unwell and breathless, and the idea or sight and smell of food upset you or make you feel ill, try to prepare your own food. Some patients (and people who do not have PAH) make meals (soups, stews) in advance and store them in the freezer ready to defrost for another day.

Fresh food, fresh vegetables, and fruit are important. Added salt is unhelpful and should generally be avoided.

Ready cooked meals

Ready cooked meals from supermarkets contain preservatives and high levels of salt and fat which, in excess, are bad for the kidneys and heart. Eaten occasionally, this is not harmful, but ready prepared meals are generally not healthy. Take-aways are convenient and better than nothing. However, they also tend to contain a lot of fat and salt, and ideally should be eaten only occasionally.

Scleroderma and the gut

Gut problems—acid indigestion and reflux, poor absorption of food, diarrhoea, and constipation—are common and a great nuisance for patients with scleroderma. It is important for them to speak to their scleroderma team about any tummy or bowel problems they have. Some patients may need high doses of antacid tablets to reduce the acid production from their stomach. If they are losing weight, this could be due to poor absorption of food and calories from the gut into the bloodstream because of overgrowth of abnormal bacteria in the bowel. Antibiotics may help this problem. Other causes of poor food absorption should also be considered, and sometimes another gut problem may need to be investigated.

Tea and coffee

Avoid excess strong caffeinated coffee and tea. It is probably better to drink decaffeinated tea and coffee to reduce the risk of palpitation due to an irregular heart rhythm caused by too much caffeine.

Alcohol

If you like alcohol, drink in moderation—no more than a glass or two of wine or half a pint of beer per day. Alcohol in low doses is relaxing and can stimulate your appetite.

Excess alcohol (more than three glasses of wine per day) can interfere with the liver and the metabolism of endothelin receptor antagonists (ERAs) and warfarin. It can make people depressed and irritate the normal rhythm of the heart, leading to palpitation and an irregular heart rhythm. This can lower the cardiac output and make patients breathless and unwell. Strong spirits are more likely to irritate the heart than wine. Alcohol is also quite fattening, and so can be a useful source of calories for thin patients, but should be reduced as much as possible if the patient is overweight.

Sex

Sex is healthy and good for you, although pregnancy should be avoided in those with PAH. The theoretical danger of sex is when patients with severe PAH strain, their cardiac output drops and their blood pressure and heart rate fall, and this can make them light-headed.

Sex is not dangerous, but how active a role you take should depend on your ability to exercise. As a general rule, if you can manage a flight of stairs without significant symptoms, anything goes, and if you are able to walk 100 metres on the flat comfortably, normal intercourse should be fine, but whatever your exercise limitation sex is safe with you playing a passive role.

Some people without PAH lose their appetite for sex as they get older. Patients with any important medical condition may also lose interest in sex and there are many reasons for this, most commonly, an anxiety or fear that sex could be dangerous.

Pregnancy and PAH

Women of child-bearing age who have PAH are advised not to become pregnant because of the very high risk to both mother and baby; 50% of mothers do not survive the full pregnancy or delivery.

Termination of pregnancy should be discussed if a patient with PAH becomes pregnant. Patients who decide to continue with pregnancy are very closely monitored, usually in hospital, and treated with disease-targeted therapies, and have a planned elective delivery.

Effective contraception using a condom is safe for the mother but not 100% effective. Progesterone-only contraceptive pills may be used.

The Mirena coil is also effective, and a combination of the oral contraceptive, a coil and the use of a condom offers the most effective contraception.

Drugs and PAH

Take the medications as prescribed. If you don't want to take them or think they might harm you, please discuss your concerns with the PAH team. If you like taking herbal or non-prescription medications, ask your PAH team if these are safe or might interact with your prescription medications. Don't stop taking your PAH tablets without first discussing this with the PAH team because your condition may deteriorate if you stop your PAH medications.

Useful contacts and PH specialist centres

Useful contacts

American PHA
850 Sligo Avenue, Suite 800

Silver Springs MD 20910

Tel: 001 301 565 3004

www.phassociation.org

British Heart Foundation
14 Fitzhardinge Street

London W1H 6DH

Tel: 08450 70 8090

www.bhf.org.uk

British Lung Foundation
73–75 Goswell Road

London EC1V 7ER

Tel: 08458 505 020

www.britishlungfoundation.com

Children's Heart Federation
Tel: 0808 808 5000

www.chikldrens-heart-fed.org.uk

Contact a Family
209–211 City Road

London EC1V 1JN

Tel: 0808 808 3555

www.cafamily.org.uk

Down's Syndrome Association

Langdon Down Centre

2a Langdon Park

Teddington TW11 9PS

Tel: 0845 230 0372

www.downs-syndrome.org.uk

Grown Up Congenital Heart Patients Association

75 Tuddenham Avenue

Ipswich, Suffolk IP4 2HG

Tel: 0800 854759

www.guch.org.uk

Heart Transplant Families Together

Wellbank

Rimpton

Yeovil, Somerset BA22 8AF

Tel: 01935 850645

www.htft.org.uk

Lupus Support Group

St Thomas' Lupus Trust

The Louise Coote Lupus Unit

Gassiot House, St Thomas' Hospital

London SE1 7EH

Tel: 020 7188 3562

www.lupus.org.uk

NHS Direct

Tel: 0845 4647

www.nhsdirect.nhs.uk

PHA Europe

www.phaeurope.org

PHA-UK

PO Box 2760

Lewes, East Sussex BN8 4WA

Tel: 0800 3898 156

www.pha-uk.com

PH Central

1309 12th Avenue

San Francisco CA 94122

www.phcentral.org

Raynaud's and Scleroderma Association

112 Crewe Road, Alsager

Cheshire ST7 2JA

www.raynauds.org.uk

Scleroderma Society

3 Caple Road

London NW10 8AB

Tel: 020 8961 4912

www.sclerodermasociety.co.uk

Transplant Support Network

23 Temple Row, Keighley

West Yorkshire BD21 2AH

Tel: 0800 027 4490/1

www.transplantsupportnetwork.org.uk

PH specialist centres in the UK and Ireland
Western Infirmary, Glasgow

Tel: 0141 211 1836

www.spvu.co.uk

Freeman Hospital, Newcastle

Tel: 0191 233 6161

Royal Hallamshire Hospital, Sheffield
Tel: 0114 271 1719

Papworth Hospital, Cambridgeshire
Tel: 01480 830541

Great Ormond Street Hospital, London
Tel: 020 7405 9200 (ext 1005/1007)

Hammersith Hospital, London
Tel: 020 8383 2330

www.pulmonary-hypertension.org.uk

Royal Brompton Hospital, London
Tel: 020 7351 8121

Royal Free Hospital, London
Tel: 020 7794 0500

Mater Misericordiae Hospital, Republic of Ireland
Tel: 00 3531 8032000

Index

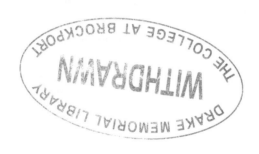